The Psychological Aspects of Intensive Care Nursing

Nathan M. Simon MD, Editor

Robert J. Brady Co.
A Prentice-Hall Publishing and Communications Company
Bowie, Maryland 20715

The Psychological aspects of intensive care nursing.

Library of Congress Cataloging in Publication Data

Includes index.
1. Intensive care nursing—Psychological aspects.
2. Critically ill—Psychology. I. Simon, Nathan M.
(DNLM: 1. Critical care—Nursing texts. 2. Critical care—Psychology. 3. Intensive care units—nursing texts. WY154 P 974)
RT120. I5P79 610.73'61 80-11365

ISBN 0-87619-663-6

Prentice-Hall International, Inc., London
Prentice-Hall of Australia, Pty., Ltd., Sydney
Prentice-Hall of India Private Limited, New Delhi
Prentice-Hall of Japan, Inc., Tokyo
Prentice-Hall of Southeast Asia Pte. Ltd., Singapore
Whitehall Books, Limited, Petone, New Zealand

Printed in the United States of America

80 81 82 83 84 85 86 87 88 89 90 10 9 8 7 6 5 4 3 2 1

This book is dedicated to Jules V. Coleman, MD

"Then felt I like some watcher of the skies
When a new planet swims into ken;
Or like stout Cortez when with eagle eyes;
He star'd at the Pacific—and all his men
Look'd at each other with wild surmise—
Silent, upon a peak in Darien."

Executive Producer: Richard A. Weimer
Production Editor: Mary Patrizio
Cover and Text Design: Marlise Reidenbach

CONTENTS

PREFACE

This book will give the nurse and other ICU professional staff the opportunity to study, in a detailed and systematic fashion, the psychological factors that have been recognized as major determinants of ICU nursing practice. It provides a framework for an orderly evaluation of the psychological issues of importance to the ICU nurse and goes on to consider the specific problems and solutions peculiar to a wide variety of ICUs. The book is meant to be practical in the best sense of the word. The experienced ICU nurses or physicians will quickly recognize themselves, their patients, and the intense work situation that is their arena of professional activity. The beginning ICU nurse or nursing student in a critical care course will be able to use the book to prepare for the actual work situation in the same way that biochemistry, anatomy, pharmacology, physiology, and ECGs are studied. The book can serve as the text for in-service seminars and for ICU staff teaching groups.

The book is written with the nurse constantly the center of focus, both as diagnostician and therapist and as subjective respondent to stress. Consideration is given in each of the chapters to the variety of psychological problems presented by patients and the complex stressful psychological and emotional world this creates for the ICU nurse. The book acknowledges the special nature of ICU nursing practice. Its intent is to share information, experience, and techniques that are related to the minute-to-minute performance of one of the most arduous and complex jobs in medicine, and it is written with the firm belief that it can contribute directly and appreciably to the ICU nurse's competence and personal job satisfaction.

The contributors to this volume are people who have all "been there" and know the issues firsthand. The glue that has bound together the views of the nurses, psychiatrists, pediatricians, psychologist, sociologist, internist, and anesthesiologist who did the writing has been the respect, admiration, and appreciation of the work of ICU nurses. It is echoed in every chapter and demonstrated by all the contributors in the sensitive, detailed attention to the personal psychological experience of the nurse. I am indebted to my colleagues for the enthusiasm, good will, and skill they devoted to this effort.

In large part, this book grew out of a personal journey of discovery—my learning experience with the MICU nurses at the Jewish Hospital of St. Louis, Missouri. They were mostly patient and tolerant teachers, who were generous in their willingness to share their knowledge and feelings and to initiate me into some of the mysteries of ICU life. Gail Poelker and Jean Parsons were especially helpful by providing the nursing care plans in this book, and Suzanne Whiteley, with her enthusiasm and advice, helped orient me at the start of my ICU work. Ruth Kelly, Medical Librarian, Jewish Hospital, repeatedly performed heroic feats of wizardry in producing references.

Finally, I acknowledge a debt to my wife and children, who exercised patience and forebearance during the time it took this book to come into being.

Nathan M. Simon

CONTRIBUTING AUTHORS

George Albertus, RN, AB, Staff Nurse, Pediatric Intensive Care Units, St. Louis Children's Hospital, St. Louis; Co-President, Hospital Staff Nursing Association.

James Billings, PhD, MRA, Assistant Clinical Professor Medical Psychology and Epidemiology, University of California, San Francisco, School of Medicine; Clinical Assistant Professor Psychiatry and Behavioral Sciences, Stanford University School of Medicine; Attending Psychologist, Department of Psychological and Social Medicine, Pacific Medical Center, San Francisco.

Neal Cohen, MD, MPH, Assistant Professor of Anesthesia and Epidemiology, University of California, San Francisco, School of Medicine; Associate Director, Intensive Care Unit, Moffit Hospital, San Francisco.

Francine Guldner, RN, BSN, Patient-Care Manager, Pediatric Intensive Care Units, St. Louis Children's Hospital, St. Louis.

Mary Brian Kelber, SN, DScN, Associate Professor, San Francisco School of Nursing, San Francisco.

Misbah Khan, Director of Pediatrics Primary Care Program; Consultant, State Department of Health and Mental Hygiene, Preventive Medicine Administration, Baltimore.

Norman B. Levy, MD, Professor, Departments of Psychiatry and Medicine, State University of New York, Downstate Medical Center, Brooklyn, Associate Editor of the *Journal of General Hospital Psychiatry*.

Gail Poelker, RN, BS, Head Nurse, Medical Intensive Care Unit, Jewish Hospital, St. Louis.

Harriet Pollard, RN, Cardiology Clinical Nurse, St. Louis Children's Hospital, St. Louis.

Patricia A. Rutherford, RN, formerly Assistant Chairman Pediatric Nursing Service, Massachusetts General Hospital, Boston.

Mary J. Sexton, PhD, Associate Professor; Director, Behavioral Science Section, Department of Epidemiology and Preventive Medicine, University of Maryland School of Medicine, Baltimore.

Nathan M. Simon, MD, Associate Clinical Professor, Psychiatry, St. Louis University School of Medicine; Supervising and Training Analyst, St. Louis Psychoanalytic Institute; Principal Investigator, Multiple Risk Factor Intervention

Trial, St. Louis Clinical Center; Consultant, Medical Intensive Care Unit, Jewish Hospital, St. Louis.

I. David Todres, MD, Director of Pediatric Intensive Care Unit, Massachusetts General Hospital, Boston; Assistant Professor of Anesthesia (Pediatrics) Harvard Medical School, Boston.

Peter Tuteur, MD, Assistant Professor of Medicine, Washington University School of Medicine, Pulmonary Disease Section, St. Louis.

Suzanne Whiteley, RN, ARRT, Pulmonary Technician, Department of Nursing, Jewish Hospital, St. Louis.

CHAPTER 1

The First Intensive Care Units: A Creative Answer Produces New Problems

Nathan M. Simon

The first nursing unit specifically identified as an intensive care unit (ICU) was a four-bed facility opened at the 180-bed Manchester Memorial Hospital, Manchester, Connecticut in the autumn of 1953. The unit was to become part of the hospital's Progressive Patient Care program, a bold plan to provide for patients specialized environments and facilities that ranged from special surveillance to self-help. In January 1954, the North Carolina Memorial Hospital, Chapel Hill, North Carolina, and the Albany Hospital, in Albany, New York, established eight-bed ICUs, and the Chestnut Hill Hospital, Philadelphia, Pa., opened a six-bed unit in May 1954. By February 1957, there were 20 hospitals in the United States with ICUs, but by May 1958, there were nearly 150.[1] In 1979, ICUs are virtually standard in the 7,000 hospitals in the United States. Major medical centers usually have several different types of ICUs within the same complex.

WHERE DID THE ICU COME FROM?

Some zealous historians would, perhaps to avoid ruffled feelings at our large, prestigious medical centers, attribute the development of the first ICU to Florence Nightingale and her ward design, which placed the sickest patients closest to the nurse's desk or in a small room immediately off of the large nursing ward.[2] It is a tribute to American individualism and creativity that ICUs began in small, nonacademic, community hospitals.

Whether or not one wishes to settle competitive feelings by attributing the origin safely to Florence Nightingale, in some ways it can be said that ICUs have been with us for a long time. The special nursing units for premature newborns, which were present many years before the first ICU appeared, meet all the criteria that are used to identify modern ICUs—critically ill patients; special facilities and equipment concentrated in these units; and specially-trained nurses using specialized nursing skills. One of the remarkable facts in the history of modern hospital development is that the basic concepts used in these highly efficient and practical premature units were not recognized as being applicable to other types of patients. The obvious benefits were overlooked until other forces in hospital patient care became operative.

Three major forces contributed to the development of the modern ICU concept. The most significant of these came from the recovery room experience that had been growing in United States hospitals after World War II. The advantage of intensive and continual surveillance of very ill patients became increasingly apparent, not only to surgeons and surgical nurses, but also to other physicians and nurses who saw the great benefits deriving from the specialized facilities and staff of the recovery room. Pressure developed to extend recovery room hours and length of stay for critically-ill patients. The identification of a group of critically-ill patients who needed special care over a period of several days rather than hours brought into being a new kind of unit that, from the beginning, differed in some ways from its recovery room progenitor.

The second major force that contributed to the development of the ICU was the progressive patient care concept, long incubating in the minds of health care planners, who envisioned a hospital in which patient groups were housed in facilities designed to meet their special needs, with the primary criteria the amount and intensity of nursing care required. Thus, intensive (two to eight hours of nursing care per day), intermediate, (two hours of nursing care per day), and self-care, (less than one hour of nursing care per day) facilities were conceived. Planners projected a number of benefits from a hospital designed to group patients in this way: (1) concentrating expensive equipment in the ICU area would bring about a substantial reduction in operating and construction costs (unfortunately, a dream never realized); (2) concentrating the most thoroughly trained nurses and ancillary personnel in the ICU to allow more effective use of their skills; (3) improving the morale of nurses by providing them with a work site that permitted them to give care needed by their patients and also to give the nurse who preferred bedside nursing to the administration of wards a place to use her skills; and (4) improving patient morale by housing them in units optimally designed to meet their needs, a goal that initially was not realized because the first ICUs, modeled on the recovery room, failed to meet the psychological needs of patients and created a group of serious problems that were unique to that design and environment. Second- and third-generation ICUs have come much closer to realizing the goal of improving patient morale.

One additional factor in ICU development was an evolving complex technology that permitted more ambitious surgical procedures (for example, open heart surgery, organ transplants, etc.) that required extensive postoperative surveillance and nursing care. Also, more intricate life supportive equipment and techniques for both surgical and nonsurgical critically ill patients became available.

In these times of $400.00 a day ICU room charges to patients, some of the earlier experiences in ICUs have a wonderful nostalgic quality to them. At the original ICU in the Manchester Memorial Hospital, the daily charge to patients was $22.00.[1] The North Carolina Memorial Hospital charged the same rate on its first ICU as the charge of the room the patient had initially occupied on admission.[3] The Rhode Island Hospital, Providence, Rhode Island, (which has the distinction of opening the first ICU housed in a space originally and specifically designed for ICU use) used the same charge policy as the North Carolina Memorial Hospital for three years, with additional costs absorbed by a special grant. Cost study at the Rhode Island Hospital in 1958 revealed that the ICU costs were actually $15.00 a day greater than the semiprivate room charge. When the hospital added this amount to the patients' bills in 1958, utilization of the ICU fell by 50%. Physicians cut their admissions to the unit because of what they felt were "exhorbitant" costs, and the surcharge was removed after a few months of near financially disastrous operation.[4]

The early ICU literature points to another factor that contributed to the appearance of ICUs in the early 1950s. This was the relative shortage of registered nurses. Some hospitals experimented with plans that attempted to provide more intensive nursing care for seriously ill patients, such as the Share-the-Nurse plan. These plans never really caught on and did little to solve the problems growing out of a need for more intensive nursing care for very sick patients. However, ICUs did appear to have an impact on the availability of nurses. For example, requests for private duty nurses exceeded the number available at the Hospital of the University of Pennsylvania, Philadelphia, Pa., by 15 to 28% in 1954, prior to the establishment of their first ICU. In 1955, the demand for private duty nurses exceeded the supply by less than 10% after their ICU had been operating for twelve months.[5]

WHAT WERE EARLY ICUs LIKE?

One of the remarkable things about the earliest ICUs, although they were developed independently in different parts of the country, was their similarity in a number of important features. The early ICUs were small (four to eight beds). They were located in quarters (most often much too small) that had been hastily converted to ICU use. Like the recovery rooms on which they were often modeled, visiting privileges were extremely limited (in recovery rooms, visiting was usually prohibited). They admitted both surgical and medical patients, but surgical patients made up about 80 to 85% of the case load. The beds were in a ward-type arrangement with individual beds separated only by curtains or screens. Equipment crowded the floor of the little space that was available. Staff learned on the job and used traditional nursing skills primarily.

The readiness of the medical and nursing communities for the ICU concept is underscored by the quickness with which ICUs changed and evolved. Some lessons were learned quickly and applied quickly. As mentioned above, the Rhode Island Hospital opened the first ICU in a working space that was specifically designed for ICU use in 1955—a 28-bed surgical ICU.[6] This unit must have been in the design stages at the time the first ICUs were opened in 1953 and 1954. It is likely that the developers of this unit were not acting on information from early ICU experience, but were applying ideas they had developed on their own. The time taken in designing a special space for this unit allowed the planners to anticipate some problems and develop creative solutions. It is instructive to examine its design for the lesson it teaches about the interaction of factors that lead to change.

The Rhode Island Hospital ICU had features that set it off from its immediate ICU predecessors and solved some of the problems of the early ICUs. This unit was specialized in regard to the type of diagnoses of the patients admitted. It only accepted surgical patients. It was a much larger unit, 28 beds all told, although these beds were arranged in four working areas. Most of the patients were housed in single rooms, all of which were under direct visual surveillance of the nurse at a central nursing station. Patient rooms had outside windows and they contained built-in oxygen, suction, and manometers. There was a room on the unit for a house officer, who was assigned full time to the unit. Special charting procedures were developed. Fairly liberal visiting privileges were permitted at staff discretion. Registered nurses assumed more complex responsibilities, some of which had previously only been performed by physicians.

In this fairly early ICU, certain features appeared that continued to strongly influence ICUs. First, the physical design was more considerate of the patient's psychological needs. The use of single rooms with outside windows is one example of this. More liberalized visiting privileges is another. Second, the scope of the nurse's activities was increased, moving into territory previously the prerogative only of the physician. Third, the unit was designed and operated so that longer patient stays could be more easily accommodated. Four, greater specialization of nursing skills was fostered, rewarded, and eventually required. There were rudiments in this early unit of a training program to equip the nurse with the special skills needed to work on such a complex unit.

Advances in medicine have brought about an increase in the numbers and kinds of ICUs. The prototypical ICU—a small unit with mixed medical and surgical patients—can only be found now in the smaller community hospital. Cardiac care units (CCU), MICU, and SICU are virtually standard in community hospitals of any size. In major medical centers, pediatric units of several types, renal units, respiratory units, burn units, neurosurgical units, and heart surgery units have been established. The trend is definitely toward more and more specialized units. The newer ICUs (renal, respiratory, pediatric, and burn units, in particular) have radically changed the focus of intensive care from acute, short-term care to semiacute and long-term care. Instead of stays of four and five days, patients on some specialized units may stay for several months. The change in the length of stay has had a profound effect on nursing staffs in the depth and intensity of nurses' relations to their patients. It also shifts the focus of psychological assessment from what needs to be done to help the patient deal with a medical or surgical crisis that lasts only a few days to a more careful, broad examination of long-standing conflicts, character traits, and social factors in the light of a progressive, constantly life-threatening illness. This is especially true if the patients are in the end stages of chronic obstructive pulmonary disease or are patients in renal dialysis units.

PSYCHOLOGICAL ASPECTS OF ICUs

The earliest discussions of psychological problems in the ICU appear to be a direct carry-over from the experience in recovery rooms.[7–10] The literature in the late 1950s and early 1960s was understandably focused on the psychological problems seen in patients in ICUs and recovery rooms. There was a running debate in the literature about the ICU psychosis or the "ICU syndrome." This syndrome was first noted in patients who were recovering from open heart surgery. The high rate of hallucinations, delusions, agitation, and confusion in patients recovering from serious surgery (which often took many hours to perform and during which long periods were spent on heart-lung machines) was noted in many papers. Efforts were also made to sort out the factors that would help in correctly diagnosing organic psychoses and differentiating them from functional psychoses. In addition, the ICU literature dealt with problems of patient survival and attempted to identify the groups of patients who had the best and worst prognoses following procedures such as open heart surgery. Finally, the literature began to pay attention to the effects of the ICU environment on the patients. This turn of events was important because it represented the first consideration of the special ICU environment as an important factor related to patient behavior and patient outcome. It became apparent rather quickly that patients on these early ICUs were undergoing a type of sensory deprivation experience.[11] The bizarre symptoms the patients presented came, in part, from being in rooms under artificial lighting 24 hours a day without awareness of the changes from day to night, from the effects of the absence of stimuli that would help the patient orient himself, such as familiar faces or clocks, and from the effects of the repetitive and sometimes disorienting noises that were part of the earlier ICUs' environment. The additional stress of life-threatening illness and painful and sometimes multiplying surgery was also recognized.

For many years after ICUs were a well-established part of hospital medical care systems, their effects on staff were overlooked, although their effects on patients received much attention. Even in the ideally-staffed ICU, which unfortunately may exist only in a table of organization that has never been adequately funded, the ICU nurse is subjected repetitively and frequently to a special set of stresses that is not part of the general nursing practice experience in general hospital wards. These stresses are: (1) constant work with a patient population that is critically ill; (2) constant work with a population that has a very high death rate; (3) emergencies occurring with great frequency, which involve life and death decisions; (4) a range of responsibility and decision-making that regular nurses' training does not equip the nurse to handle; and (5) caring for patients, sometimes for weeks or months, who are maintained by mechanical life support systems, where decisions about continuing or discontinuing these support systems are daily occurrences.

The ICU differs from the usual nursing unit not so much in the uniqueness of any one single feature but because of the frequency with which these experiences occur on the ICU. The quantitative change from general nursing practice is so great that it produces a working environment qualitatively different.

There are recurrent themes in the early ICU literature that are concerned with the nurse, the scope and nature of her role, and her morale. Predictions were made early that the ICU would be beneficial because it would improve nursing morale.[12,13,14] The possibility that the ICU would create new problems for nurses was not foreseen by early ICU advocates and, once ICUs were established, there was a slowness in recognizing the presence of these problems.

The issue of nursing morale is a complex one. It will be considered in detail in the chapters of this book. The chapters that follow will take up the special environment in a variety of ICUs. The features of different types of ICUs will be examined in detail. The primary focus will be on the psychological aspects of the nurse's practice. This focus includes a consideration of the working environment, the character of the patient population, the psychological responses of patients to the ICU, the ways in which the nursing practice situation produces a range of psychological responses in nurses, and, finally, ways in which the psychological problems the nurse must deal with in her patients and herself can be identified, diagnosed, and treated.

SUMMARY

The factors leading to ICU development in the United States were: (1) recognition by nurses and physicians of the advantages to patient care that were possible in the surgical recovery room; (2) a long-standing interest by hospital planners in developing hospitals with graded areas of patient care; and (3) advances in medical science that allowed new procedures to be performed and that spurred the development of new medical technology. Early ICUs were greeted with enthusiasm because of predicted benefits to patient care and nursing morale. Unfortunately, no one predicted that ICUs would have inherent within them forces that can lead to significant disruptive problems for patients and nurses. Patient problems were recognized and responded to relatively quickly, but there was a lag of nearly 15 years before the seriousness of the stress of ICU nursing practice was recognized.

REFERENCES

1. Golin M: At Last—A Hospital To Fit Doctor-Patient Needs. JAMA 166: 2180–2183, 1958

2. MGH News, Boston, April 1969, p. 2

3. Cadmus RR: Special Care For The Critical Case. Hospitals 28: 65–66, 1954

4. Olsen HV Jr.: Are Specialized Units The Answer To Better Patient Care and Lower Costs, Unpublished Presentation At Mid-Atlantic Hospital Assembly, May 21, 1959

5. Last T: Concentrating On The Critically Ill. Mod Hosp 86: 69–72, 1956

6. Beardsley JM, Bowen JR, Capalbo CJ: Centralized Treatment For Seriously Ill Surgical Patients. JAMA 162: 544–547, 1956

7. Blachly PJ, Starr JA: Post-Cardiotomy Delerium. Am J Psych 121: 371–375, 1964

8. Kornfeld DS, Zimberg S, Malm JR: Psychiatric Complications of Open Heart Surgery, N Engl J Med 273: 286–292, 1965

9. Abram HS: Adaptation to Open Heart Surgery: A Psychiatric Study of Response to the Threat of Death. Am J Psych 121: 659–668, 1965

10. McKegney FP: The Intensive Care Syndrome: The Definition, Treatment and Prevention of a New Disease of Medical Progress. Conn Med 30: 633–636, 1966

11. Solomon P, Leiderman PH, Mendelson J, et al: Sensory Deprivation: A Review. Am J Psych 114: 357–363, 1957

12. Sandove MS, Cross J, Higgins HG, et al: The Recovery Room Expands Its Service. Mod Hosp 83: 65–70, 1954

13. Bell, E: Special Nursing Unit Relieves the Strain. Mod Hosp 83: 74–75, 1954

14. Wagner, RA: How Does the Intensive Care Unit Affect Nursing Morale and Utilization. Nursing Outlook 6: 286–288, 1955

CHAPTER 2

Psychological Assessment: Gathering Data

by Nathan M. Simon

Hospital Patient Revolts: Takes 2 Others Hostage

Baltimore (UPI)—Cardiac patient Carroll Davis saw one patient in his hospital room die Friday morning. Then he saw doctors struggle with a spinal disease patient resisting an injection. He decided he had had enough.

Davis ripped the intravenous tubes from his arms, ran out of his room in the Intensive Care Unit of University Hospital, and barricaded himself and two other patients in a semiprivate room down the hall, police said.

Spokesman Dennis Hill said Davis held the patients for six hours, until he was assured of a television interview.

"It was a combination of stress and his illness that caused him to undergo temporary insanity," said Dr. Thomas Ducker, Chief of Neurosurgery at the hospital.

"He was in a room with one patient who had died earlier in the night, another awake with a spinal disease, and a third acutely ill patient next to him."

"The doctors at the time were with a patient on his left and gave her a needle in her back to get a brain fluid sample," Ducker said. "That patient resisted, and to Davis it looked like they were trying to kill her."

The two barricaded in the room with Davis were freed by police, while Davis was granted a short television interview by station WJZ-TV in a hallway, Hill said.

He said Davis had watched television coverage of the incident and agreed to surrender if the station would interview him.

Hill said neither Davis nor the post-operative brain surgery patients with him suffered any harm from the ordeal.

Deborah Ross, 26, one of the patients locked in with Davis, said Davis was very frightened.

"When he first came in, he shut the door and dumped water on the floor, then grabbed me and shoved me in the chair," she said.

"He then broke a window, but when he saw the 12th floor was too high to jump from, he sat down. After a while he became peaceful and very nice," she said.

Davis, who had been under observation for chest pains for about 72 hours before the incident, was returned to the intensive care unit under supervision.

"We were concerned that Davis may have had a heart attack during the incident," Ducker said.

Hill said he did not know if Davis would be charged.[1]

The psychological aspects of the ICU inevitably become a matter of importance for all of the people—patients, families and staff—who are part of the ICU. It is a part of the total clinical situation that must be carefully identified, understood, and dealt with in ways that will serve both the best interests of the patients and the nurse's role as an effective professional. The nurse who does not evaluate the psychological elements runs the risk of being caught up in uncontrolled ways in psychological conflicts. Understanding psychological factors gives the nurse the perspective that can make possible the optimal use of nursing skills in each patient's cause. It also provides insights that lead to creative adaptations to the stresses that are part of the working life on the ICU.

All patients who come to an ICU must be seen in a psychological framework, but not necessarily as "psychiatric patients." To view someone in a psychological framework is to recognize that the person: (1) is more than a disease or a diagnosis (not just the "MI in room 478" or the "acute leukemia in room 1106"); (2) has a set of needs, motivations, and feelings about self and others that influences behavior; (3) influences and can be influenced by people; (4) has a reaction to the illness that brought about admission to the ICU; and (5) has a history of living and adapting to the world, and that the characteristic style of adapting will probably become apparent in the ICU environment.

There are a number of reports in the scientific literature from both clinical and experimental studies that emphasize the importance to the nurse of the psychological factors in ICUs. Animal experiments by Richter,[2] Lown,[3,4,5] Taggart,[6] and Skinner[7] have established the role and mechanism of psychological stress in the production of arrhythmias leading to sudden death. Papers by Lown,[8,9,10] Harvey and Levine,[11] Rahe and Christ,[12] Engel,[13] Cannon,[14] and Taggart[6] have described the relation of psychological stress to cardiac death in man. These reports describe cases of ventricular arrhythmias of various types (VPCs, tachycardia, fibrillation) induced by psychological stress.

Jarvinen[15] described a particular type of psychological stress related to the ICU. He found a relationship between sudden cardiac death and ward rounds by the physician-in-chief of a cardiac unit. Some of these deaths were in patients expecting to be discharged on the day of the ward rounds.

A number of papers provide cogent support for special attention to emotional issues on ICUs. Vreeland and Ellis[16] described nurses on a SICU stressed by the following situations: (1) feelings of inadequacy in dealing with obtunded patients; (2) difficulties in maintaining objective attitudes towards patients in extreme pain. The nurses experienced conflict because of the need to be firm and objective and at the same time exhibit warmth and feeling; (3) inappropriate sympathy by nurses, which eventually leads to a withdrawal from the patient; (4) high expectations from the medical staff about performance and attitudes; (5) the stress of decision-making related to situations where the choice lies between calling the physician immediately or deciding that the call to the physician can be postponed; (6) problems in caring for very regressed and dependent patients. The nurses must be adequate to accept the regression initially. There must also be readiness to teach and lead the patient to greater independence and to avoid the temptation of saving time by "doing it herself"; and (7) lack of quiet time to reflect on her work.

Hay and Oken[17] described stresses on ICU nurses because of: (1) repeated exposures to death and dying, leading to feelings in the nurse of threat of loss of important people and a sense of personal failure; (2) defensive distancing by the nurse to solve an immediate feeling problem that frequently creates the secondary problems; (3) lack of gratification from obtunded patients and from work overload that leads to trouble in maintaining self-esteem; (4) the specialized nature of the work leading to communication breakdown with doctors, families, and nursing and hospital administrators; and (5) the necessity of very close group cooperation that leads to increased intragroup tension.

Kaplan De-Nour[18] described how nursing practice on renal dialysis units leads to feelings of guilt, possessiveness, overprotectiveness, and withdrawal from patients. Staff often reflect unrealistic wishes that the patient do extremely well on the treatment program and at times deny that the patient is ill. Also, there are frequent differences between physicians and nurses about how they view the patients. Physicians on these units often see the patients as suffering less and nurses often view the patients as suffering more. Kaplan De-Nour[19] has described how team opinions about patients develop. There is generally more agreement in terms of the patient's physical condition and less agreement about the amount of suffering a given patient is experiencing. Nurses are consistent in their distortions of a given variable and will tend to see all patients in somewhat the same way. These discrepancies highlight the presence of nonobjective personal bias that influences the way a patient will be treated.

Dubovsky[20] and colleagues, in the only controlled study of the effectiveness of psychological approaches to problems of ICUs, have demonstrated that regular use of psychiatric consultants and group meetings for ICU nurses resulted in a decrease in death rate in the experimental unit. That decrease was only in the rate of acute cardiac deaths. They also found increased efficiency in charting in the experimental unit and increased time spent by nurses with their patients. It also appeared that the nurses on the experimental unit were more sensitive to the situations that may have triggered fatal arrythmias in their patients. The experimental unit appeared to be calmer and more efficient with the higher degree of open communication.

Cassem and Hackett[21] surveyed CCU nurses to identify areas of stress. The nurses mentioned conflicts with nursing administration as the largest source of stress, with scheduling and staffing, families of patients, research procedures, other nurses, patients, and physicians following in order of decreasing concern. They found considerable anger, depression, frustration, and anxiety related to the concerns, which had considerable impact on their unit morale.

Gentry[22] compared the responses of nurses practicing in ICUs and in general medical surgical wards of a university medical center to a battery of psychological tests that measured depression, anxiety, self-concepts, hostility, and guilt. He found, in general, that ICU nurses reported more depression, hostility, and anxiety than non-ICU nurses. There were differences in guilt, self-esteem, and personality pattern. The psychological responses appeared to be associated with situational stress, including overwhelming work load, too much responsibility, poor communication between nurses and physicians, limited work space, and too little continuing education.

The response of the already overworked ICU nurse to a suggestion that she perform yet another task could understandably be an exasperated groan. But there is reason to temper that response. First, the primary purpose of psychological evaluation must be functional. The question must always be "What do I need to know to help me deal in the best way with my patient?" A corollary question which often provides the most critical part of the answer is "What do I need to know about myself and my feelings?" Second, the information needed is almost always readily available and often obtained without special effort by nurses in their regular bedside contacts with patients or in their contacts with the patient's family. Third, the psychological evaluation process can lead directly to nursing care plans that make the nurse's practice more effective and reduce the tension growing out of feelings of anger, frustration, and helplessness.

The purpose of the psychological assessment of patients admitted to an ICU is to mobilize the maximum resources available to help the patient deal with a serious life-threatening illness. It will identify the psychological strengths that can be brought to bear effectively in the crisis the patient is living through. It also will identify the psychological liabilities that may seriously impede or interfere with the patient's most effective treatment. In the crisis-filled minutes and hours of ICU work, only those issues immediately pertinent and functional need to be considered. For the patient admitted to an ICU in an acute crisis, a set of priorities develops out of that immediate crisis. For the patient with a semiacute or chronic illness or the patient who will have a longer stay on the ICU, there will be other priorities developed, sometimes much more far-ranging in scope.

The method of data collection and the type and amount of data collected for psychological evaluation may look formidable as it is described in these pages. How much is needed at any given time during an ICU stay will vary widely from patient to patient. However, the method of assessment is the constant that provides access to what is useful. A functional psychological evaluation should produce a psychological nursing care plan that is a part of the overall nursing care plan. In the best of working conditions, this plan should be developed logically after the necessary data collection has taken place and be written as part of nursing notes so that it will be immediately available to all nursing staff caring for the patient.

There is much value in writing out the psychological nursing care plan. It can lead to clarification of ideas and problems, move away from vague and hazy suggestions about what should be done, and reduce failures in accurately conceptualizing the issues that must be dealt with. Where written nursing care plans are not done routinely, psychological nursing care plans should be discussed at nursing report shift change and at rounds with medical staff.

GATHERING BASELINE DATA

Nurses often accurately appraise the psychological elements in the clinical situation intuitively. The intensity and complexity of clinical issues in an ICU suggest that there is a need to go beyond this intuitive evaluation to a systematic one that can be shared with the rest of the staff. A systematic psychological evaluation and the development of the psychological nursing care plan grow naturally out of the methods that the nurse routinely uses to assess the physiological parameters in her patients.

The same sources of data are available. For a physiological evaluation, the nurse makes use of direct observations (vital signs, color, breathing pattern, motor behavior of the patient, etc.), patients' reports on their condition (pain, discomfort, itching, bloating, cramping, dizziness, feeling hot or cold), indirect observation (family reports of patient's behavior, patient's history, lab reports, etc.). Some data gathered either directly or indirectly can be immediately interpreted and become the basis for an initial treatment plan. However, other data can be useful only if they are compared to data about the patient's condition prior to the time the patient was admitted to the ICU. This is to say that baseline information can be essential in making sense out of any single set of observations about a patient at a given time.

Baseline data are most easily obtained when the patient is admitted in a steady psychological state that causes no concern about psychological issues. Any deviation can be then compared against reference points that have been built up in first-hand contact with the patient. The immediate importance of baseline psychological data is more apparent when the patient arrives in a state that causes concern about psychological functioning. For example, a patient is admitted with labile affect, cries easily, and moves rapidly from a joking conversation to marked open anxiety. In order to make an accurate assessment of this behavior, it is necessary to know how characteristic it was of the patient prior to the patient's admission to the ICU. Similarly, it is needed for evaluations of patients who are mostly silent, patients who are angry or demanding, patients who are depressed, or patients who are hallucinating.

Baseline data are also valuable in assessing the clinical importance of the patient's response to the ICU itself. It is an axiom of ICU experience that the conscious patient first admitted to an ICU will have some emotional response to: (1) the stress of the serious illness that brought about admission; and (2) the new and strange environment of the ICU. This latter factor is especially important for elderly patients, who may have chronic brain syndrome, and for children. Both of these age groups are most sensitive to changes in the physical environment and respond with disruption of functioning.

The patient's responses to other major crises in life can be compared to the behavioral response to admission. The patient or the family may be able to say that "X always cried at times like this" or "Y always minimizes his pain" or "Z always ignored what the doctor said just to prove he was tough" or "A always acted dumb and never seems to understand what people tell him."

If a patient, who is described by the family as a reserved, quiet person, is effusively talkative and reveals intimate personal details of his life after admission to the ICU, it is important to recognize this as unusual behavior that probably indicates a high level of anxiety. It would be a mistake to identify this as a mark of trust and confidence in the nurses to whom it is displayed.

An important component of data gathering for the psychological evaluation is learning about what the patient was like before he became ill, and, if the illness has been lengthy, what he was like during the period of his life immediately prior to the ICU admission. The following areas should be evaluated when possible:

1. The patient's prevailing temperament and mood. Had the patient been characteristically friendly or seclusive, angry, challenging, open, private, domineering, helpless, depressed, indecisive, pessimistic, or optimistic?

2. The patient's characteristic coping mechanisms. What are the ways in which the patient characteristically deals with other illnesses and stresses in his life? Does the patient respond realistically or ignore, deny, minimize, become depressed or angry?

3. The patient's level of intellectual functioning.
4. The patient's knowledge about his illness.
5. The patient's social class and ethnic group.
6. The patient's family constellation. It is important to know which people are closest to the patient; the number of his or her children and siblings; whether the patient's parents are living; whether there have been any deaths or serious illnesses in the family.
7. Recent events in the patient's life that may have a bearing on the patient's attitude toward his illness. Has the patient had a recent success or difficulty on a job, has the patient recently retired, has the patient suffered a financial reversal, has someone close to the patient moved away or returned after an absence?

Where can the baseline data be obtained? The sources are normally readily available from: (1) the patient; (2) the patient's family; and (3) the patient's chart, which may contain information from previous admissions or workups done on other divisions of the hospital. At shift change report, information gathered by several nurses who have had contact with the patient and the patient's family members can be shared. This offers an excellent opportunity to collate baseline data. Ward rounds with the medical staff is another important source for gathering and collating data about the patient's condition prior to admission to the ICU.

There are some patients for whom baseline data are difficult to come by. Examples are elderly patients who have no close family or who are transferred from nursing homes, or patients of any age where the family is not available because of geography, working conditions, or emotional reasons that lead to avoidance. However, in these situations, if baseline data are necessary, efforts to contact sources of information can be initiated by the physician, the nursing staff, or the hospital social worker. This sometimes will mean a telephone call to families that live at some distance or the more active pursuit of family members by the staff of the ICU in order to talk to them about the patient and get the information that is necessary for assessment.

GATHERING IMPORTANT CURRENT DATA ABOUT THE PATIENT

We know and understand our patients in many ways quickly and intuitively and form impressions about them, sometimes in the first few minutes of contact, that may last for the entire time we work with the patient. We gather information without being aware of it. It's only when we are required to identify where our global responses come from that we trace the sources of the data that lead to those responses. The following section contains a guide for a systematic survey of factors, which provides us with input to permit assessment of our patients. It includes a list of things that we routinely observe and catalog. This helps us identify the interplay of the psychological currents that are active during the patient's ICU stay.

Facial Expression

The observation of the patient's face provides quick information about emotional state. Moods and feelings—depression, elation, pain, anger, fear, bewilderment, worry, annoyance,—all are often discernable. The type and duration of eye contact provide clues to the quality of contact that the patient is able, at that moment, to establish with us. Patients may try to avoid emotional contact with nursing staff by "looking through" them as if they are not present or by looking over the head of, or to the side of, the nurse. The face turned away—turned to the wall—is often a graphic acting out of hopelessness and despair.

Motor Behaviors: Body language, mannerisms, tics

Observation of motor behavior yields information of two types. The first type is expressive in a general way of affect or feeling tone. Behavior of this type is the clenched fist of unspoken anger or the rigid body that expresses anxiety or fear; the movement toward or away from a nurse or a visitor that is an expression of the wish to be closer or the wish to escape contact; the reaching out of hands that is an expression of the wish to make contact, be cared for, comforted.

The second type of observation is used in making more formal psychological diagnoses. In this category are such things as the motor retardation that is characteristic of depression; hyperactivity in mania; catatonia or waxy flexibility in schizophrenia; tics in some neuroses; paralysis, agitation, aimless picking, tremor, and athetoid movements that are present in organic brain disorders.

Speech

The style, rate, quality, and content of speech all offer information about the patient's emotional state. The style of speech often depends on regional or dialectical conventions. However, within any dialectical subgroup, individual characteristics are discernable that indicate deviation from the norm and give clues to the emotional state. Mumbling, whispering, drops in volume in mid-sentence or at the end of sentences, and loud expletives are examples. Archness, coyness, secretiveness, suspiciousness, superiority, arrogance, pretentiousness, or humor are qualities that can be expressed in the style and vocabulary of a person's speech.

Rapid speech is often associated with anxiety, and more extreme forms can be seen in conditions like mania. Very slow speech is frequently seen in organic brain syndromes, depression, and some psychoses. Total absence of speech is characteristic of organic brain syndromes and certain severe psychotic conditions. Blocking—that is, stopping in mid-sentence—is often evidence of an inward state of distraction. This also can be produced by anxiety and in some cases of organic brain syndrome.

Content of speech can be examined in several ways. The appropriateness of speech is an important area to evaluate. Speech can be evaluated for the way in which it expresses an accurate appraisal of what can be consensually validated. The structure of logical thought patterns is expressed in speech and accessible to evaluation. Speech can be studied for the presence of nonsense words or newly invented words. Speech also can be evaluated in the degree to which it matches the speaker's observable feeling state as demonstrated by how the speaker looks or the emotions that are displayed. Speech can be understood in the ways that it is used indirectly to plead, frighten, command, seduce, distract, shock, or intimidate the listener.

It is useful to remember that speech, regardless of its content, is one of the most frequent ways of making contact with another person.

Thought and Intellectual Functioning

Thought patterns are usually evaluated by observations of the patient's speech, but can be evaluated by writing or gestures in patients who cannot or will not speak. The capacity of the individual to think in a logical style in the usual sense of cause and effect reasoning should be appraised. It is important to note the organization of what is said. Sometimes ideas will be expressed in sentences that are confused, poorly constructed, and grammatically illogical. Individual sentences may be well constructed, but they may be illogically connected to one another. It is valuable to determine how effectively the speaker can pursue an idea to its goal. Some speakers will avoid pursuing a thought to its conclusion by changing the subject and still others will flood the listener with so many details that the point is never reached. When such behavior occurs, attempts should be made to assess whether it is a specific idea or subject that produces the behavior or whether it is a long-standing characteristic of the patient with all subjects and ideas.

Assessment of memory, both recent and long-term, can be done easily and naturally in the discussion that goes on with the conscious patient on admission. Patients with chronic brain syndromes often show recent memory impairment while retaining good memory for distant events. If there are gaps in recent memories, especially in the events related to the patient's illness, those should be noted because often they deal with events and feelings that the patient finds too painful or stressful to deal with. Some patients with memory gaps will attempt to fill them by "making up events" (confabulation). This is seen most often in organic brain syndrome. It is valuable to know if the patient is aware of memory deficits. Awareness of deteriorating memory can be extremely painful and the source of great humiliation to patients.

Judgment

Poor judgment can produce grave consequences when the patient embarks on some course of action that has been forbidden by medical orders or if the patient fails to report a change in physical condition. The nurse can accumulate information about the conscious and speaking patient's ability to make reasonable, sound judgments in the discussion she conducts during the admission procedure. Determining the level of comprehension and understanding can be one of the more difficult tasks for an ICU nurse, as speech may be interfered with by shifting levels of consciousness, intubation, or tracheotomy. It is usually most directly evaluated as the nurse asks the patient to follow simple instructions. More complex and abstract levels of understanding that involve complicated ideas and subtleties of feeling and mood are more difficult to determine then. There is often a considerable difference of opinion among nursing and medical staff about a patient's ability to comprehend. When this occurs, it is useful to discuss the differences in a conference and, if necessary, request consultation with a psychiatrist or a neurologist.

Nurses are remarkably innovative in working out simple communication systems with patients who are unable to speak because of mechanical obstructions such as intubation. These spontaneously devised communication systems will provide clues to understanding. Working with a written notes system, a system of eye blinks and nods, or lip reading with patients can be a slow, painstaking procedure. It is important for the nurse who is trying to evaluate the patient's understanding and judgment not to jump hastily to conclusions and especially not to put words or ideas into the patient's mouth. The wish to have an understanding and communicating patient can often lead the nurse to fill in for the patient whose ability is absent or compromised. This can lead to an overestimation of the patient's ability to understand—a problem common enough among relatives of critically ill, partially-conscious, patients and one best not added to by the nursing staff.

Comprehension and understanding are related in part to the patient's intelligence. Some estimation of intelligence is necessary to provide perspective about the patient's ability to make judgments. However, comprehension can be markedly interfered with by shifting levels of consciousness, pain, medications, brain oxygenation, and anxiety so that even very bright people under the impact of severe illness and the ICU environment might appear to be relative dullards.

There is a deeply ingrained force that makes some physicians and nurses treat every person in a hospital bed as if his or her intelligence level was below the age of eight. Patients, even very sick patients, including young children, for that matter, react negatively to the condescension they sense in the "talking to the child" type of communication from medical or nursing staff. There is also a problem at the other end of the spectrum. Sometimes nursing staff will only be comfortable using highly technical terminology. Most often, the nurse who does this attempts to avoid communicating openly and honestly with patients and/or is avoiding some painful feeling. Language that is too technical will result in explanations that are beyond the patient's level of true understanding. Knowing the patient's educational level, listening to the patient's own vocabulary, knowing something about the patient's social background will all be useful in helping determine the most useful way to go about explaining things to the patient.

Quality of Relations with Self and Other People

The nurse's frequent contacts with the patient and her ability to observe the patient's interactions with family and other hospital personnel provide an almost endless series of opportunities to evaluate the way the patient feels about self and other people. Serious illness almost always produces a centering of attention on oneself and a microscopic concern and interest in one's body in all aspects of its functioning. There is often an expectation that others should be, and are, concerned in the same way. This attitude is normative behavior in the ICU setting, and it is reinforced by the medical and nursing staff's continual interest and questioning about the patient's condition. However, some people have this characteristic of heightened self-centeredness as a central feature of their personality. Any threat to body integrity, function, and appearance can be a source of extraordinarily intense anxiety, depression, or anger for people like this. All serious illness, whether mutilating surgical procedures or illness involving nonvisible internal organs such as hearts or kidneys, can produce the sense of threat to body integrity and appearance.

In order to evaluate the feelings the patient has about self and the quality of relations with other people, there are a number of questions the nurse can ask herself as she works with a patient:

1. How sturdy and stable does the patient's sense of self-worth and self-esteem appear to be? Is there some ability of the patient to like him or herself?

2. Does the patient have a sense of self as an independent, separate person? The stress of life-threatening illness renders many people transiently dependent and clinging. Such individuals, for short periods of their hospital stay, appear to be unable to do even the simplest of things by themselves and seem to require someone in the room with them constantly. However, for the majority of individuals, this represents a fleeting set of behaviors. In others, it is a stable character trait that may have been present long before the illness and hospitalization.

3. Does the patient see options or personal resources that are available to deal with future life situations? Patients who see themselves without options for leading useful lives often develop severe depressions that interfere with treatment on the ICU and their rehabilitation afterwards.

4. Does the patient regularly voice self-critical or self-depreciating thoughts? Does the patient blame everything that goes wrong on other people or on the hostile and unfriendly world? The latter group of people often sees the nursing staff and medical staff in a rather suspicious way. While apparently cooperating with medical and nursing regimens, they may be involved in hidden campaigns to subvert the people who are caring for them because they see them as controlling authorities. Self-depreciating, self-critical patients may be masking hostility as well as demonstrating a lack of self-esteem.

5. Does the patient show a capacity for objective self-observation? Patients who are able to see themselves accurately, including the sometimes silly or unreasonable ways in which they behave, are in a position to be much better allies with nursing staff in their treatment programs. Also, people who have this capacity for self-observation generally will demonstrate some sense of humor, some ability to laugh at themselves, as well as at others.

6. In what way does the patient regularly relate to other people? Does the patient adopt a straightforward attitude of trust that permits working together? Can the patient allow enough dependency behavior to be appropriately cared for? Does the patient remain distant and uninvolved or suspicious? Does the patient present a passive, infantile helplessness or an angry, demanding, frightened claim for attention? How much controlling and demanding behavior is exhibited? What happens to the patient's anxiety level when alone or in the presence of others? Does the patient show preferences for (or show marked differences in behavior with) either men or women, doctors or nurses, older, the same age, or younger people? Similarly, does the patient seem to behave differently with people to whom he feels superior than to people he considers his inferiors?

Affects, Feelings

The optimally functioning nurse will observe and respond therapeutically to the emotions expressed by patients. The starting point for evaluation of emotions considers the type of feeling and whether it is appropriate to the situation. In addition, the appropriateness of the feeling to the patient's verbal and nonverbal communication should be considered. Other aspects to be evaluated are the intensity of the emotion and how long it lasts. Different ethnic groups and cultures permit, encourage, or discourage expression of specific emotions. This must be considered in evaluating the patient's emotional state.

Some concern should be given to whether or not the patient struggles to avoid expression of emotions. Sometimes this is done out of shame or out of a wish to protect others. Some patients feel that the expression of certain emotions, especially negative feelings, is unacceptable and they try never to give voice to these feelings.

The constant monitoring of emotional state in patients and in oneself can be a trying and painful process. It leads to a gold mine of information, but it is hard, hard work. At times, nurses block out or turn away from their patient's emotional state because accurate recognition yields a level of distress that is not personally acceptable at that time. This can be highly selective and individualized. The nurse on a given day may not be able to acknowledge anger expressed by a patient. Or, similarly, a nurse may turn away from jealousy and competitive feelings expressed by a patient. A not uncommon situation is the conscious patient who is dying and aware of his condition. Such a patient sees the nurse as the person who will go on living and often expresses jealousy and resentment about this. Also jealousy and resentment are often demonstrated when the nurses and the patients are about the same age and sex and the patients see themselves as not able to do the things the nurse can do. Another common situation is intolerance of and failure to recognize the extreme states of helplessness and despair of patients who are beyond help. This is because it touches on the nurse's own helplessness and is a threat to her professional identity.

Sometimes an emotion can be used to mask or exclude another emotion. Patients may use anger to avoid fear, depression to avoid anger, or hypomania to mask depression. Apathy, hopelessness, and severe depression are especially important emotions of which to be aware because their presence has grave prognostic implications. Patients who exhibit this triad of feelings need to be considered for carefully worked out nursing plans because so many of them do not survive. Depression and anxiety are affects that are present almost universally. When they are not present, some thought must be given to accounting for their absence.

NURSING CARE PLANS

Below are three examples of psychological nursing care plans. They are reproduced as written by nurses on an MICU. The information about diagnosis, age, and complication has been added to make the nursing care plan intelligible.

---

1. White Jewish male, age 57, Ph.D., university professor, first MICU admission. Antero-septal MI and pericarditis.

NURSING CARE PLAN

Problem	*Plan*
Anxious, fearful—expresses fear of death, concerned over absence of teaching duties.	Encourage verbalization of fears and questions. Explain procedures. Give answers as possible. Refer to

Problem	Plan
	physician when needed—accept him.
Family also fearful.	Explain all procedures. Answer questions, if possible.
First hospitalization. Concerned about loss of privacy.	Close door. Cover him up when possible. Explain necessity when privacy sacrificed.

---

2. White Protestant female, age 96, widow. First MICU admission. Acute pulmonary edema. Rule out MI.

NURSING CARE PLAN

Problem	Plan
OBS—disorientation.	Orient frequently to place and situation with special emphasis on where and how to call the nurse.
Hard of hearing.	Speak slowly and distinctly; get return of information.
Almost blind.	Identify yourself when entering room, touch frequently. Explain set-up of room. She listens to TV. Explain trays and help.

---

3. White Protestant female, age 85, housewife, married, four grown children. MI. Cardiac Arrest. Cardiac Tamponade. Intra-arterial blood pressure—left femoral artery. Arterial line right radial artery.

NURSING CARE PLAN

Problem	Plan
Semicomatose—responds to pain stimuli.	Explain all procedures in simple terms and with brief explanations. Orient patient to person, place, time, situation of shift, and as frequently as possible. Have doctors address pa-

Problem	*Plan*
	tient when in room. Talk to patient during AM care. (Can include time of year, weather, news events, etc.) Encourage MDs to explain treatment and patient's progress. Be honest with patient.
Pain—discomfort due to ET tube, balloon pump, Swan Ganz, arterial line.	Observe for signs that patient is having pain, restlessness, diaphoresis, etc. Give pain meds as ordered. Orient patient to tubes and reason for them.
Altered level of consciousness (physiologically induced. Maybe experiencing delusions, hallucinations.	Expect fear of death, pain, altered body image, loneliness (in addition to Nursing Orders for Problem #1). Talk to patient in calm, soft voice. Touch is important! Move and touch as gently as possible. Encourage patient's family to hold her hand and talk to her. Family may bring radio and set station patient has liked in past. Play for a few intervals throughout day as patient tolerates.
Family's fear of equipment, loss of loved one with critical illness.	Keep informed of progress, encourage questions. Answer questions, using calm, clear, simple explanation. Refer to House Officers.

Each of the three nursing care plans identifies specific problems and, in most instances, outlines actions the nurse can embark on to effectively deal with the problem. The first example, however, illustrates how nursing care plans can omit precise prescriptions for the nurse. "Encourage verbalizations" might be made more specific by describing how the nurse could accomplish this. (Respond verbally and nonverbally with positive statements or gesture at those times when the patient begins to talk about his fears; be unhurried and calm when the patient begins to talk about his fears; ask nonthreatening questions about the patient's fears, indicating interest in what the patient has to say; empathize with the patient about the understandability and appropriateness of his fears; ask the patient about questions and concerns at times when he does not verbalize them spontaneously.) Similarly, translating "accept him" into specific activities could be spelled out for this patient. (Cultivate a calm, unhurried attitude while the patient is talking about his anxieties; show positive feelings and interest in all his questions; avoid any hint of evoking criticism or shaming behavior when the patient talks about his anxieties; make visits to the patient's room at times other than when the patient calls for assistance; sit quietly with the patient at times when he is not especially talkative.)

The nursing plan should lead to clarifying the nurse's activities even if, in some cases, it means doing nothing—for example, not responding when the patient discusses certain subjects or sitting with a patient as time allows without carrying out any procedure. The illustrations are offered, not as ideal examples, but as typical of those written by nurses on a busy ICU who are aware of their usefulness.

SUMMARY

Well-documented animal and human studies have demonstrated the importance of psychological factors for both patients and nurses in the ICU. Accurate psychological assessment is necessary for the highest level of nursing practice. Psychological assessment must be related to both the immediate and long-term needs of the patient, and selectivity is needed to make the type of evaluation done fit each clinical situation appropriately. Gathering information about the patient's psychological functioning prior to his hospitalization, as well as baseline psychological data immediately after admission, helps in assessment of the emerging patterns of feelings, behaviors, and symptoms. Suggestions are made for gathering and utilizing key information about the patient's facial expression, motor behavior, speech, intellectual functioning, judgment, quality of interpersonal relations, and feeling states. The value of a written nursing care plan that focuses specifically on the psychological aspects of the patient is emphasized.

REFERENCES

1. Reprinted by permission of United Press International

2. Richter CP: On the Phenomenon of Sudden Death in Animals. Pyschosom Med 19: 191–198, 1957

3. Corbalan R, Verrier R, Lown B: Psychological Stress and Ventricular Arrhythmias During Myocardial Infarction in the Conscious Dog. Am J Cardiology 34: 692–696, 1974

4. Lown B, Verrier R: Neural Activity and Ventricular Fibrillation. N Eng J Med 294: 664–665, 1976

5. Lown B, Verrier R, Corbalan R: Psychological Stress and Threshold for Repetitive Ventricular Response. Science 182: 834–836, 1973

6. Taggart P, Parkman P, Carruthers M: Cardiac Response to Thermal, Physical and Emotional Stress. Br Med J 3: 71–76, 1972

7. Skinner, JE: Theories of the Frontal Cortex in Regulation of Cardiac Vulnerability to Ventricular Fibrillation: A New Concept of Cannon's Cerebral Defense Mechanism in Neuro Physiology and Psychology. *In* Donchin B, Gailbrath G, Kaetzman M, (eds): Basic Mechanisms and Clinical Application, Academic Press, 1979

8. Lown B, Reich P: Ventricular Fibrillation and Psychological Stress. N Eng J Med 294: 1347–1348, 1976

9. Lown B, Tempte JU, Reich P, et al: Basis for Recurring Ventricular Fibrillation in the Absence of Coronary Heart Disease and Its Management. N Engl J Med 294: 623–629, 1976

10. Lown B, Desica RA, Lenson R: Roles of Psychological Stress and Autonomic Nervous System Changes in Provocation of Premature Ventricular Complexes. A J Card 41: 979–985, 1978

11. Harvey WP, Levine SA: Paroxysmal Ventricular Tachycardia Due To Emotion. JAMA 150: 479–480, 1952

12. Rahe RH, Christ AE: An Unusual Cardiac (Ventricular) Arrhythmia In a Child: Psychiatric and Psychophysiologic Aspects. Psychosom Med 28: 181–188, 1966

13. Engel GL: Sudden and Rapid Death During Psychological Stress: Folklore or Folk Wisdom? Ann Intern Med 74: 771–782, 1973

14. Cannon WB: Voodoo Death. Psychosom Med 19: 182, 1957

15. Jarvinen KAJ: Can Ward Rounds Be Dangerous To Patients With Myocardial Infarction. Br Med J 1: 318–320, 1955

16. Vreeland R, Ellis GL: Stress On The Nurse In the Intensive Care Unit. JAMA 208: 332–334, 1969

17. Hay D, Oken D: The Psychological Stresses of Intensive Care Unit Nursing. Psychosom Med 34: 109–118, 1972

18. Kaplan De-Nour A, Czaczkes JW: Emotional Problems and Reactions of the Medical Care Team in a Chronic Hemodialysis Unit. Lancet 2: 987–991, 1968

19. Kaplan De-Nour A, Czaczkes JW: Professional Team Opinion and Professional Bias—A Study of a Chronic Hemodialysis Team. J Chron Dis 24: 533–541, 1971

20. Dubovsky S, Getto CJ, Gross SA, et al.: Psychiatrists on the Coronary Care Unit. Psychosom 18: 18–27, 1977

21. Cassem N, Hackett TP: Sources of Tension for the CCU Nurse. Am J Nurs 72: 1426–1430, 1977

22. Gentry WD, Foster SB, Froehling S: Psychological Response to Situational Stress in Intensive and Nonintensive Nursing, Heart Lung 1: 973–976, 1972

CHAPTER 3

Psychological Assessment: Frequently Seen Syndromes and Defenses

Nathan M. Simon

The discussion that follows will focus on the patient and the nurse within an adaptive framework. The language is often from the domain of psychiatry and psychology. While this is in large part a product of the author's training and practice, it is also used to introduce frequently used concepts in a language known and used by ICU professionals. The emphasis is *not* on psychopathology. The psychological terms used are not judgmental nor invoked to "label." The people—patients, nurses, physicians—coping with the special set of stresses will remain in the center of the stage. The language and diagnostic process are intended to provide an entry into the complex human interactions that are characteristic of ICU environment.

Information about human behavior and feeling can be organized in a number of different ways. The alternatives that lead to effective action will be given primary consideration here. Most of the examples used not only illustrate some aspect of coping by a patient or nurse, but also indicate a statement of the effectiveness of the action and sometimes offer suggestions for alternative courses of action. In a very action-oriented profession, as is nursing, it is sometimes difficult to immediately become aware of the benefits derived from purely internal processes, such as correctly sorting out and identifying the components in one's own feeling state in relation to another individual (patient or staff) that do not immediately lead to some physical act. The internal, sorting-out process may eventually make it possible for the nurse to say something to a patient about his (the patient's) fear of dying, or apologize to a colleague for an unwarranted accusation about not sharing responsibility, or initiate a conference with the nursing office about correcting an intolerable staff shortage.

Many times internal evaluations lead to rather subtle changes or actions and may make it possible for a nurse to stay in a room with a patient who was previously visited only perfunctorily, or to respond without rancor or anger to demands or threats by a patient, or to clarify and clearly set limits with the patient about what kinds of behavior are acceptable. Evaluation done alone and shared with others often allows for new ways of perceiving both oneself and the other person involved in a complex interaction.

Human conflict and human crises must first be perceived before appropriate action can be developed. For a nurse to walk by a weeping patient without interest or inquiry would, to present an exaggerated example, be a statement that categorizes the patient as a "nonproblem" and a "noncrisis." Second, the nature of the problem in terms of the individual at that particular moment in life needs to be elucidated. The patient in the example above could be weeping for joy, sadness, pain, anxiety, anger, or relief. To elucidate accurately requires using what is already known about the patient and often involves inquiries to discover what elements that were initially unknown may be playing a part in the situation. Third, nursing activity to help the patient resolve the conflict or reduce the stress engendered by the conflict is chosen on the basis of the best understanding of the origins of the problem and the resources of the patient and staff. There is a wide range of activities that are employable—education and clarification, simple and direct reassurance, environmental manipulation, interpretation, empathic understanding, encouragement of expression of feeling, discussions of areas of concerns previously off limits, behavior modification techniques, (positive reinforcement, shaping), "proper distancing," programs of planned activity, involving the family (or disengaging the family), discontinuing or initiating medication, changes in staff caring for the patient—these are some of the activities frequently initiated and carried out by the ICU nurses.

There is one final point that deserves emphasis. Not all problems are "solvable" in the usual sense of the word, which implies improvement, success, or tension reduction. There are situations in which the short-term resolution may contain little or nothing that speaks of success or tension reduction. For example, after the unexpected death of someone much loved it may only be after a period of mourning that takes months to accomplish that significant tension reduction is achieved.

Similarly, failure to obtain a deserved and desired position can produce feelings of anger and frustration long after the event. Some personality conflicts are not resolvable with mutual good feelings resulting on everyone's part. Some unfair and unsatisfactory administrative policies are not amenable to change even by the most dedicated and sincere efforts. Some patients will not respond to even the most thoughtfully conceived and faithfully executed care plans.

To distinguish what is changeable from what is not is, in itself, a critical task that offers some protection against the pitfalls of either the extreme position of omnipotence or the extreme position of helplessness when confronted with an initially puzzling, serious, and complicated clinical or administrative problem.

ANXIETY

Hackett[1] has identified anxiety as the most frequently experienced emotional state of patients on a coronary care unit (CCU). While there are no comparable quantitative data for other types of ICUs, the author's observations lead him to believe this holds true for all ICUs who admit acutely ill, as well as fully conscious, patients. The identification and management of anxiety becomes an important issue for ICU personnel.

Anxiety is the feeling state that accompanies awareness of danger. A small amount of anxiety is called signal anxiety and usually leads to a response that reduces or does away with the dysphoric state. However, in circumstances in which the individual has attempted to cope and failed, is further overwhelmed by stress, and/or is unable to call forth any adaptive and defensive responses, the anxiety state may persist and be experienced as almost unendurable.

Some differentiate anxiety into responses to a real external danger and responses to an internal, unreal (neurotic) danger. In the ICU, the combination of real and unreal dangers is ever present. To be anxious (afraid) about dying before open-heart surgery or kidney transplant would be an example of a predominantly real external threat. To be anxious on being left alone in a hospital room for 15 minutes three days after surgery and in the course of an uneventful recovery would be an example of predominantly internal danger. The more internal "unreal" threats are prominent, the more anxiety is considered maladaptive and a sign of psychopathology.

Neurotic anxiety is the unresolved residue of responses to danger situations that is part of the normal developmental sequence. From a developmental view, neurotic anxiety was at one point in time a reaction to a "real" danger situation. These normative developmental experiences are fear of loss of sense of self; fear of separation from important nurturing protecting figures; fear of loss of love and fear of subsequent disapproval and criticism; fear of loss of control; and fear of damage to the body. The qualities that distinguish neurotic anxiety are: (1) the anxiety is often displaced to an object or situation that is not the real source of the anxiety (phobias are examples of this); and (2) the amount and intensity of the anxiety is not appropriate to the stimulus that triggers it. The critical developmental issues that are normal sources of anxiety in infancy and childhood are readily reactivated by serious illness and hospitalization even in people who had adequately resolved them earlier. This accounts for the ease with which the fears of the real dangers associated with admission to an ICU can be amplified, intensified, and prolonged, as they are reinforced by anxiety from the experiences of early life.

Anxiety, as a signal, has an adaptive purpose. It evokes maneuvers by the individual to avoid a dangerous situation and the intense physiologic discomfort and helplessness that accompanies the fullblown anxiety state. Signal anxiety attached to too many important social and interpersonal situations becomes maladaptive because, while the primary danger may be avoided, defenses that appear in response to the signal exact a debilitating toll in themselves. Overwhelming anxiety and diffuse, unfocused chronic anxiety are evidence of failure of signal anxiety to evoke adaptive mechanisms.

Helplessness-hopelessness can be described as an end stage of extreme anxiety and depression. Schmale[2] and Engel[3] have identified these states as components of the "giving up" complex, which has a grave prognostic implication. Helplessness-hopelessness develops when the individual is stressed either actually or symbolically and perceives an inability to cope with the stress. Helplessness-hopelessness in an otherwise physiologically well-functioning individual can be part of the etiology of a physical disease. In the already physically sick individual, it may play a critical part in a downward course that leads rather quickly to death.[4,5,6]

Anxiety is a subjective state—an intrapersonal internal experience, but one with objective signs. Increased pulse rate, rapid breathing, cold, sweaty palms, transient increases in blood pressure, evidence of muscular tension, and "cracking" of the voice are frequent signs of anxiety. In addition, there are other signs or symptoms that may appear, such as GI symptoms (nausea and vomiting, diarrhea, belching), increased frequency of urination, sleep disturbance, motor restlessness, faintness, blushing, or pallor. In extreme anxiety states, an individual may be virtually frozen and unable to act or speak.

The subjective experience may range from slight uneasiness through apprehension, the anticipation that terrible things will happen, a feeling of doom and/or panic that one is going to be completely overwhelmed.

Valium has almost become part of standing orders for patients admitted with myocardial infarction to CCUs and for many patients on other types of units. Anxiety management, however, must go beyond the routine administration of a tranquilizer. For many patients on MICUs, respiratory units, SICUs, and neurological units, tranquilizers of any sort, major or minor, are contraindicated because of side effects such as depression of the respiratory center, effects on cardiac rhythm, vagus stimulating effects, and clouding sensorium.

In these situations, anxiety reduction and management is a matter exclusively between and among people. It has been a well-established medical fact for over two thousand years that a competent, calm, understanding, empathic human being can be a reliable and effective tranquilizer and the one with the fewest undesirable physiological side effects.

There are a number of ways in which a nurse can effectively reduce patient anxiety. The most frequent general anxiety-reducing behavior is the calm, interested, helpful presence of the nurse who listens empathically and who may hold the patient's hand or perform some routine act such as adjusting a pillow, providing a drink, or giving a bed bath. The nurse, without being interpretive or even talkative, by her physical presence and nonverbal behavior can greatly reduce patient anxiety. In this sense, the nurse serves to evoke the calming and healing memories of adequate mothering that took place in the earliest years of life.

Anxiety reduction can be enhanced by careful understanding of the patient's view of the hospital experience. Nurses who take time to answer questions carefully and thoughtfully and explain procedures in detail to the patients before initiating them can reduce anxiety appreciably.

Anxiety reduction can result from the nurse's ability to serve as a model for the patient by indicating a readiness to talk about painful, frightening, or shameful concerns. The nurse can indicate by her strength and openness that it is possible to give voice to feelings of despair or hope; to be able to talk about death or life; to cry without shame. Patients gain courage and strength from nurses who are able to recognize and facilitate the need to talk about subjects usually barred from polite conversational interchanges.

Another key to anxiety reduction in the ICU involves accurate identification of the sources of the anxiety. The anxiety may involve something specific like the patient's response to forced inactivity, to a concern about a particular relationship with family or staff, to overdependence on a mechanical support system (ventilators, monitors). This type of anxiety reduction usually can be provided only after careful listening, sometimes with the assistance of a consultant, and the assembling of facts so that a logical therapeutic approach is possible.

For some specific anxiety situations, a behavioral approach is possible. Plans can be initiated to systematically avoid reinforcing specific patient behaviors that are dysfunctional. Examples are: being disinterested if the patient discusses a subject that always produces unwanted increases in dependence behaviors; going into the patient's room before the patient pushes the call button so as to interfere with the patient's developing a strong connection between pushing the call button and the appearance of the nurse. Systematic desensitization can sometimes be accomplished and, on occasions, simple relaxation techniques can be taught.

There are situations in which the nurse's ability to take a firm, positive stand will, in the long run, turn out to be anxiety-reducing. Many patients work themselves into anxiety states as they attempt to test limits to see if they can either avoid a situation they find distasteful or get more control over the people who are caring for them. When this is the case, "giving in" tends to have a somewhat paradoxical result in that the patient's anxiety becomes greater. There are sometimes prompt and marked decreases in anxiety when the nurse is able to clearly, and without being angry, set limits and make it clear that the procedure will be carried out in ways that are necessary.

DEFENSES AND COPING MECHANISMS

The awareness of anxiety produces adaptive maneuvers the purpose of which is to decrease the amount of perceived anxiety and to work out a compromise within the individual about the conflict or crisis that triggers the anxiety. Most of the adaptive process takes place unconsciously. In the following section, a group of these coping mechanisms will be illustrated, first in a general way and then with some specific examples from the ICU.

In order to describe defenses and coping mechanisms, it will be useful to use a hypothetical situation.

A very large and hungry-looking lion enters a room in which a man is sitting.

Repression

If the man reacts by saying the room is empty, he is utilizing *repression. Repression* occurs when a perception is refused both preconscious and conscious registration and mental representation. *Repression* is a defensive maneuver that is perhaps the most frequently used defense because—while it is usually not seen in its pure form as in the illustration given here—it works in combination with other types of defenses to block from awareness some critical element that gives rise to conflict and anxiety.

Regression

If the man were suddenly to defecate, urinate, begin crying for his mother, or flailing his arms about, he would be demonstrating *regression. Regression* is adopting feelings, behaviors, and thought patterns characteristic of an earlier stage in development.

Intellectualization

If the man moves toward the exit door and begins calmly talking about the dangerous situation he is in, including the observation that he is frightened, he is using the defense of *intellectualization. Intellectualization* is the accurate recognition of a threat of a conflict—an accurate description of the emotion appropriate to it. However, there is no evidence that the man is actually experiencing the emotion that he says is appropriate to the situation.

Isolation

If the man moves toward the door after calmly noting that the lion is hungry and dangerous, but expresses or describes no feelings at all, he is demonstrating the defense of *isolation*, in this case of feeling, and, of course, *repression* as well. Isolation is the separation of feeling and idea (conscious thoughts) and the barring from consciousness of one of the elements—the feeling state.

Denial

If the man were to make no attempt to leave and were to prepare to eat lunch, and, if asked about the situation, would correctly describe it—that is, the man would be able to say that the lion is large and very hungry-looking and that the lion might indeed at any moment eat him—he would be using *denial*. *Denial* is a coping maneuver in which there is correct recognition of a danger situation or feeling but in which the person fails to accurately work out the implications that grow from the perception. That is, while the man correctly identifies the dangerous situation he is in, he does not draw from it the proper conclusion that he should change his course of action radically—to leave or to try to defend himself against the lion's attack. It is important to understand the meaning of the defense and coping mechanism of *denial*, which is different from the usual dictionary use of "denial," which means to "declare not to be true" or "refusal to grant."

Displacement

If the man were to begin to talk about how frightened he was of having a toothache, he would be using *displacement*. *Displacement* is a coping maneuver in which feelings appropriate to a situation are experienced and recognized by the person in the situation. However, because the situation is so conflicted, it cannot be correctly identified, and the person attributes the feeling to something or someone other than the actual source.

Regression and Counter-phobic Behavior

If the man reacts by saying he likes nothing better than to fight and defeat a hungry lion and if he rushes barehanded to attack it, he is utilizing *regression* and *counter-phobic behavior*. The *regression* is demonstrated by the appearance of behaviors and thinking patterns characteristic of an earlier stage in psychological development. In this example, it is regression to omnipotent thinking. *Counter-phobic behavior* is doing what one is most afraid of. In the example, the fear of being attacked by the lion is replaced by statements of pleasure and attempts to attack the lion.

Projection

If the man were to say the lion was very frightened of him, he would be using *projection*. In *projection* one attributes an internally perceived feeling state or wish to someone or something outside himself.

Identification

If the man were to leave the room promptly, suddenly find himself hungry for some fresh raw meat, and enter a restaurant to eat steak tartare, he would be using *identification* to cope with the stressful situation. *Identification* is modification of oneself to take on the characteristics and qualities of another.

Sympathy

If the man, while still in the room, were to become overwhelmed by sorrow and carried away by tears about the plight of lions who are kept in captivity and not fed properly, and because of his tears were to make his escape impossible or difficult, he would be demonstrating *sympathy*. *Sympathy* is feeling sorry for someone's plight. There is a direct involvement in the situation in which one's own feelings are as important as the feeling of the person who is in difficulty. This confuses one's role and does not allow appropriate action because of the failure to maintain a sense of discreetness and individuality.

Empathy

If a man, after promptly escaping, were to call for help in capturing the lion and, after the capture, help feed it, and then talk about how he understood that lions became hungry and that it was a problem for them (even though he did not care to satisfy the hunger by becoming the main course of a lion's dinner), he would be demonstrating *empathy*. *Empathy* is the accurate and sensitive perception of how someone else feels, while at the same time retaining one's identity, not confusing one's role, and allowing one to act in the appropriate way.

CLINICAL EXAMPLES

Repression

A 59-year-old divorced man with advanced invasic and metastatic lung cancer kept asking the house officer why they were keeping him in the hospital and what was wrong with him. They had, on several occasions earlier in his hospital stay, explained that he had a tumor or a growth. The house officers requested a psychiatric consultation. During the interview with the patient, the psychiatrist told him he had cancer of the lung, that it had spread to several parts of his body, and, while the physicians could give him some treatment to help with the symptoms, the outlook was grave. The next day, and for the remainder of his hospital stay, the patient complained to the house officers and the nurses that no one had ever told him what his diagnosis was or why he was being kept in the hospital. This patient used repression very promptly to keep the diagnosis from his consciousness as it was too threatening for him to be able to deal with it openly.

The nurses and physicians were understandably responding to their own distress at the patient's use of repression in such a flagrant way. The attempts to get him to give up this defense were resisted quite successfully by the patient. The best course at that point would be one that did not further challenge the patient. The nurses who cared for him could empathize with his complaints at not being told his diagnosis and the reason for his hospitalization. They could refrain from challenging him, they could be interested in what he thought was the trouble, and they could empathize with him about the situation of being ill, having painful treatments, and not showing any improvement. Most of this behavior could be described as an attempt at relationship building. It would also have been useful to use the same nurses on each shift as much as possible to provide care for the patient in order to assist in this relationship-building plan. Because the man had led a lonely and isolated life, the nurses should not attempt to become too close or too friendly, but should give him the distance that he appears to have always needed in order to maintain some degree of stability.

Repression and Denial

A 3-year-old boy with severe congenital heart disease underwent corrective surgery during which he suffered severe brain damage and did not recover consciousness. By the end of the first postoperative week, the mother had accepted the situation and was talking openly about the impending death of the child. The father never talked openly about his son's hopeless situation. Every day he would visit and question the nurses to see if various procedures were being carried out. His behavior unnerved the nursing staff. They appealed to the neurologist, who rather abruptly confronted the father. The neurologist said to the father, "You must know your child will die soon." The father's response was "Does that mean that, if something comes up so that you can help my child, you will not?" The physician again explained the hopeless situation. This time the father replied, 'You take care of my child and let me take care of myself." After the child's death a few days later, the father began to grieve appropriately. During the first postoperative week the father was not able to deal with his feelings about his son's impending death. In order to support himself in that position, he primarily utilized repression and denial.

In this situation, the doctor's authoritarian confronting manner completely ignored the father's emotional response to the crisis of his son's impending death. The nurses and doctors themselves were in some ways very caught up in the tragedy. Perhaps they somewhat overidentified with the mother and were angry at the father for not demonstrating the feelings they thought were appropriate and to be expected of someone whose son was about to die. The author's recommendation would have been for the nurses and physicians to have talked over the situation initially before attempting to confront the father. Such a discussion might have clarified some of the nurses' and doctors' angry feelings toward the father that were inappropriate and that did not recognize the fact that the father had a psychology of his own that he was using to try to protect himself. It could have been useful to have the nurses and physicians available to the father as he requested, to answer questions directly and honestly without elaboration or trying to force the father to "accept" the implications of the answers, and to recognize empathically with the father that his son's grave and hopeless condition was an almost indescribable blow. This approach could have been taken in ways to avoid intruding aggressively into the father's defensive position at a time when he clearly indicated that he was not ready to mourn openly and needed more distance and time.

Isolation, Identification, and Projection

A 38-year-old man was admitted to a neurological ICU immediately after automobile accident in which the car he was driving struck a bridge abutment. His wife and two young children were killed in the accident. The patient's only complaint was a headache. After several days, the medical and nursing staff became concerned because the patient showed no grief, even though he talked about the accident with those who questioned him. The nursing staff's primary concern was that the patient would commit suicide. It appeared that the nursing and medical staff were projecting the guilt they would have felt in that situation about the deaths of the wife and children onto the patient and expecting him to act in a suicidal way out of grief. It is also possible that, for some staff, the concern about suicide represented a way of dealing with their anger toward the patient. For these individuals, the equation was "I wish I could punish him by killing him because he killed innocent people. That thought is not acceptable; therefore, he should commit suicide." The patient's history revealed that he had always been a distant man, never involved in close emotional relationships with anyone, including his family. He also was a person who, throughout his life, had never shown feelings. His headaches cleared up in a few days. He had an uneventful course after discharge. The patient was predominantly using isolation, as he had for most of his life.

Regression

A 61-year-old, married, childless woman was admitted to an MICU for the second time in six weeks with a myocardial infarction. Before becoming ill, the patient was a fastidious dresser who spent much of her time in grooming herself in order to present a modish and youthful appearance. Her husband was interested in her appearance and supported her in these activities. On her first admission, which was also for an MI, she made herself up elaborately, sometimes with her husband's assistance. She would not let the nurses wash her face for four days because she didn't want to ruin her eye makeup. She was active and did as much as she was allowed to do during this stay. She had an uneventful course. She was readmitted shortly after discharge with a second MI and in congestive failure. A tracheotomy was performed in the Emergency Room because of severe respiratory distress. Physiologically, the patient stabilized quickly. This time, however, there was a tremendous anxiety and she was unable to use the defenses that had helped her on the first admission. On the second admission, she lay inert, would not care for herself, would not move herself or even swallow. She constantly used the call light to summon nurses. It was only after a great deal of difficulty and with many feelings of anger evoked in the nurses who cared for her that the patient began to gradually resume activities that involved self-care.

A nursing plan that considered the patient's great involvement in her appearance and body (her narcissism) might have been helpful. The nurses could have attempted to separate their appearances in the patient's room from the call light by coming frequently for short periods of time before the patient had a chance to call for them and by letting her know specifically when they would return. The times could have been lengthened gradually. In some ways, this would have been seen as a shaping technique, with frequent visits being the operant, and letting the patient know that the nurses' reappearance was in some ways contingent on the patient's waiting for the required time. At the same time, specific, positive comments about her appearance could be made. The use of cosmetics could have been introduced as early as possible. The patient's husband's aid could have been enlisted by discussion with him alone about the problem and what he could do to help it. He could have been encouraged to make specific positive comments about the patient's appearance and to offer to help her with her makeup, as he had often done in the past. Because the patient's demandingness created such anger in the nurses, switching nurses frequently could have been considered here until the time that the patient's demandingness decreased.

One other course of action could have been considered. Some verbalization with her about her feelings of anger and resentment at being let down so completely and having to return to the hospital so soon after her initial admission could be attempted.

Denial

A 65-year-old married man was admitted to the CCU for the first time with a diagnosis of myocardial infarction. The patient was anxious for several hours on the first hospital day. His chest pains disappeared rather quickly with the use of morphine. He was told he had had a heart attack, but that it was not large and that he would do well. His vital signs stabilized rather quickly. For the remainder of his four-day stay, he was cheerful and optimistic and talked about all the things he would do after discharge.

As long as the patient participated in his treatment in an appropriate way, the nurses need not take any course of action that would run afoul of the patient's denial. The patient could have been involved in the early phases of an education and rehabilitation program. The nurses could have reinforced his optimistic positive outlook while, at the same time, specifically reinforcing him in areas in which he was following courses of behavior that contributed directly to his recovery and also to lowering his risk of another heart attack.

Denial and Displacement

A 45-year-old married man was admitted to a CCU with a large myocardial infarction. He had several episodes of arrhythmias with significant drops in blood pressure and spent ten days in the CCU. He was an extremely bright man who knew a good deal about medicine through extensive reading. Prior to his transfer to a regular nursing division, he had been given extensive information about his illness in the educational rehabilitation program for patients with MI. When he was transferred to his new room on a regular nursing division, the window was open at the top and it was cool in the room. The patient called the nursing station on the intercommunications system and asked someone to close the window. It was about 45 minutes before an aide came to his room. She found that he had pushed a heavy three-drawer dresser to the window, put a stool on top of it, and was in the process of climbing up on the furniture to shut the window. When questioned, he said he knew about the risk he was running in doing what he did and that someone with a recent heart attack should not do much vigorous physical work. But, since no one had come and it was very cool, he thought it was better that he close the window. He was much more concerned about the coolness in his room than the possible effect of the physical exertion. Later, when talking with his physician, the patient was able to say how angry he was that no one came promptly and that he was anxious about being transferred from the security of the CCU, where help was always available. This patient, in addition to using denial about the consequences of his behavior, also displaced his primary concern about being left alone and in circumstances where he felt much more vulnerable onto his concern about the temperature in the room.

Several possibilities were available to ameliorate this problem. Early discussion with the patient about transfer would have been useful. Reassuring him that the ICU nurses would follow him to the general medical floor and visit him regularly there could have been of some help. Greater interest in the patient's anxiety about his illness could have been possible if not quite so much emphasis had been initially placed on his intellectual mastery of his illness. There were, of course, management errors when he was transferred to the general medical floor. Better communication between the ICU staff transferring the patient and the staff of the nursing floor could possibly have reduced some of these problems. The floor to which he was transferred could have been told about his anxiety and suggestions could have been made about frequent visits to the room during his first few days of stay on that floor. If this course of action had been instituted, his anxiety and anger about transfer may have been shifted to less dangerous courses of action. The other issue that comes up with this patient relates to whether or not his nurses and physician had identified the problem as being so severe as to make psychiatric consultation a useful adjunct to his treatment.

Projection, Displacement, and Regression

A 70-year-old white male had been on the unit for several days. It became necessary to intubate him. The patient was extremely restless and in poor contact. He extubated himself several times. He was finally restrained. After one of the times he extubated himself, the patient told the nurse that he felt someone was trying to put a tube down his grandson's throat and that he was trying to protect his grandson. The nurses found that sitting with the patient and quietly talking to him calmed him down considerably and decreased the patient's restlessness and attempts to extubate himself. When the patient improved, his tube was removed and he had no memory of ever being tubed.

The nurses found the correct intervention for this patient very promptly and carried it out in an excellent way. Staying with the patient proved to be a very effective way of reducing his restlessness and anxiety and cut down on his efforts at extubating himself. Haloperidol might have been considered to help the patient over the initial phase of his agitation.

DEPRESSION

Depression is a feeling state and a diagnostic category. Hackett found depression to be the second most prevalent emotional state in CCU patients.[1] In units where patients have longer stays, depression is ubiquitous and the major psychological problem. It is rare to find a patient on an RICU, a Burn Unit, or a Dialysis Unit who does not have some depressive symptoms. Depressive symptoms can be primary in the sense that the patient had them prior to the illness resulting in ICU admission. Depressive symptoms can be secondary in the sense that the patient developed them in response to the emotional meaning of the illness that caused admission or that they are the product of the physiological changes of the illness itself. As with anxiety, there are mixtures of these options frequently seen on ICUs.

Depression is one of the most frequent responses to loss—loss of self-esteem, control, important other person, nurture, love, body part, power, independence, or a viable future. There are other dynamic issues intimately involved in the appearance of depressive symptoms. One of these is anger. In some depressions, there is considerable internalized and self-directed anger. Related to the anger is marked ambivalence to important figures whose actual or threatened loss or withdrawal of support precipitate the depression. The ambivalence and the feelings of a dependence on important others combine to make direct expressions of anger impossible. At the same time, guilt feelings and self-reproach are spin-offs from the internalized anger.

Illnesses that result in ICU admissions are, unfortunately, excellent breeding grounds for depressions. They almost always involve one or more of the losses mentioned above and gain added strength from pre-existing problems around identifications with important, ambivalently-held, people. The nursing staff frequently are treated by patients as if they were the important people in the patient's life and they become the target for the ambivalent feelings.

Depressive symptoms, like anxiety, can have an adaptive function for adequate psychological resolution of the experience of loss. Depressive symptoms are characteristic of both normal mourning and pathological depression. Criteria that distinguish mourning from depression are: (1) length of time symptoms persist; and (2) appropriateness and extent of responses. One must attempt to distinguish between the two states in order to develop a useful treatment plan. Empathic responses that acknowledge that a loss (of a body part or function) has taken place and that a grieving period is necessary and expected are the correct and supportive ways of dealing with the normal mourning experience involving serious illness.

The signs of depression are depressed-looking faces, tearfulness, motor retardation (occasionally there is agitation instead), insomnia (early morning awakening is characteristic of more serious depressions), weight loss (sometimes in milder, more chronic, depression weight gain is seen), preoccupation with death and dying, self-critical statements, and suicide attempts or suicidal thinking.

Symptoms of depression are decreased self-assurance, decreased sexual interest, decreased appetite, (sometimes its opposite—there is an increase in appetite and constant eating instead), constipation, loss of initiative, decreased energy, constriction of interests, lack of pleasure from usually pleasurable activities, and overall pessimism. Chronic fatigue and chronic pain are often considered to be depressive equivalents.

In short stay ICUs, and especially with first admission patients, the nursing approach involves sorting out depression from mourning, and, if depression is identified, protecting the patient and beginning the work of recognizing with the patient the factors related to the onset of the depression. Also, where it is consistent with the overall medical regime, nursing care plans that encourage and support early activity and that are aimed at early education and rehabilitation are valuable. There is some evidence that suggests that initiating psychotherapy during the earliest days of hospitalization cuts down on posthospitalization disability in patients with MI.[7] On longer stay ICUs, more definitive treatment plans need to be implemented. These may include psychotherapy and/or the use of antidepressant medications if they are not contraindicated. (See papers by Klien[8] and Jefferson[9] for a good review of side effects of antidepressants.)

ACUTE AND CHRONIC BRAIN SYNDROMES AND SCHIZOPHRENIA

Major psychiatric disturbances are not infrequent on ICUs. In the earliest days, when ICU patient populations were largely made up of postcardiac surgery patients who had spent long periods on heart-lung machines and when the design of ICUs maximized patient disorientation and confusion, psychotic episodes were so common that the term "ICU psychosis" became a popular diagnostic label. It's striking how little one hears this term now. The nursing staff of an ICU develop a high level of tolerance for bizarre psychological behavior. Psychiatric consultations are rarely used for the "run of the mill" organic psychosis. Most often, the credo appears to be "Let's work around this as best we can, as long as it doesn't interfere with other treatments."

The three diagnostic categories that appear with some frequency on ICU—and often cause difficulty in correct identification because their symptoms and signs are often overlapping—are: (1) chronic brain syndromes; (2) acute brain syndromes; and (3) acute psychotic reactions (schizophrenia). There is clinical value in making a differential diagnosis correctly because treatment plans that relate to each of these syndromes are somewhat different. In chronic brain syndromes, the treatment emphasis will be in maximizing orientation, providing familiar faces, avoiding medication that diminishes or clouds consciousness, and maximizing activity. In acute brain syndromes, the control and careful protection of the patient during the most disturbed part of the episode, directing efforts at removing the cause, and withholding medications that will depress the sensorium are important. In acute or chronic schizophrenia, the use of anti-psychotic drugs, efforts to deal with the patient's suspiciousness, understanding the patient's symbolic communication, and beginning psychotherapy promptly are all important early treatment measures.

Good history taking is often critical in distinguishing among these three entities. In early chronic brain syndrome, the history often reveals an elderly person who is functioning fairly well in his home environment but who begins to show florid signs of disturbance when admitted to the hospital. Another variant of this picture is the elderly individual, functioning at home at an adequate level, who develops intercurrent illness with fever, infection, or congestive failure, and suddenly begins to show areas of impairment and deficit prior to being hospitalized. History of acute brain syndrome reveals an individual who had been functioning fairly well prior to the disturbance but with evidence of some acute toxic condition—the ingestion of large amounts of toxic substances such as bromides, barbiturates, or alcohol, or some major physiological insult such as stroke. In schizophrenic illness, there is usually a history of major chronic psychiatric disturbance beginning early in life and a history of psychiatric treatment (use of major tranquilizers and psychiatric hospitalization).

As mentioned above, it is often difficult to separate these syndromes and there are frequently mixed pictures—quite commonly an acute brain syndrome superimposed on a chronic brain syndrome or an elderly schizophrenic with a chronic brain syndrome. The table on pages 54 and 55 summarizes the major features of these syndromes.

AMBIVALENCE: THE PATIENT AND THE MACHINE

Ambivalence is the presence of contradictory and opposing thoughts and feelings about the same person, object, or situation. The love-hate relationship of the patients to the complicated surveillance and life-sustaining machinery to which they are attached is complex and often has far-reaching implications for the treatment and rehabilitation plans. The first machine to become important in ICUs was the cardiac monitor. In the early ICU experience, an impression grew among some workers that patients were upset by the cardiac monitors and made anxious because of the visual and auditory reminders of heart action. Interviews with patients, however, revealed that in recent years nearly 90% are either reassured by the monitor or are neutral to its presence.[1] The approximately 10% who dislike the monitor are impervious to explanations about its usefulness.

The other two machines that are frequently part of a patient's ICU experience are the ventilator and the hemodialysis machine. Attitudes to both are more openly ambivalent. Patients frequently gave nicknames to hemodialysis machines, which indicates both their dependency on them and their anger at and fear of them. Anxiety about machine malfunctioning is high, especially in the early stages of hemodialysis. The marked ambivalence to the machine and the dialysis itself is demonstrated by the frequency with which it is part of suicidal acts. Patients who exsanguinate deliberately are known to every dialysis unit.

Ambivalence to the ventilator is equally marked and open. It is complicated because the ventilator deprives patients of the ability to communicate easily. Patients who are intubated while conscious are subjected to great physical discomfort. The dependency problems that develop during extended periods of assisted ventilation can be difficult to deal with. The patient who usually hates the ventilator at the same time often becomes frightened when it is either turned down or off. The anxiety produces respirations of poor quality, which worsen the problem and lead to greater need for ventilator assistance in maintaining blood gases at functional levels.

GUIDELINES FOR TALKING WITH PEOPLE WHO ARE PATIENTS

Everyone is, at the very least, a secret psychologist. Despite disclaimers and protests of professional innocence, a little talk about human problems will reveal strongly-held convictions and theories about what "makes people tick" and, if they are not "ticking" properly, what can be done to get them to do so.

Self-conferred expertise in human psychology, publicly proclaimed or secretly held, has understandable roots. Much of it comes from the propensity all of us have for examining our own thoughts and feelings. As far as we know now, this is one of the unique characteristics of homo sapiens. Most of the time we believe we "know" how our minds work and why we act and feel as we do. Reinforcement of our self-conferred expert status takes place easily as we transfer to it the power we have from areas in which we have genuinely earned our spurs as nurses and doctors.

Personal convictions about human psychology are both a blessing and a burden. At times they can, almost magically, allow us to appreciate and understand the nature of another's inner experience. Accurate understanding can lead to appropriate, therapeutic, human responses. We use it to know when to be silent, when to protect, when to be firm and insistent, when to acknowledge a painful feeling, and when to encourage and support.

At other times, we interpret psychological phenomena mostly or wholly on the basis of our own needs. When this occurs, our interpretations run a great risk of being inaccurate, a barrier to understanding, and of little use in leading us to helpful therapeutic responses.

Formal training in talking with people who are patients does not play a significant part in the nursing undergraduate curriculum. Some time is devoted to communication theory, the nurse-patient relationship, and psychiatric diagnoses. Little or no time is spent teaching and supervising nursing students in skills of communication as a therapeutic modality.

Talking to people in such a way as to understand and help them is an art and a skill. Nearly everyone can learn how,

TABLE 1. ***Characteristics of Chronic Brain Syndrome, Acute Brain Syndrome, and Schizophrenia.***

	CBS	*ABS*	*Schizophrenia*
Type of onset	Usually gradual, but florid picture can appear with new environment or sudden illness	Usually sudden	Variable
Age of onset	Usually later life	Any time, but elderly more susceptible	Usually late adolescence or early adulthood
Emotions	Labile, irritable	Apprehensive, irritable, agitated	Flat, inappropriate
Personal appearance	Careless	Careless	Usually careful
ORIENTATION			
Time	Early; usually only slightly impaired—can be fluctuating	Markedly impaired to absent	Good (when testable)
Place	As above	As above—usually mistakes unfamiliar for familiar; i.e., hospital is home	Usually impaired, and when impaired is bizarre; i.e., "I am on Mars"
Person–Self	Unimpaired	Unimpaired	May be impaired; i.e., "I am Jesus"
Other	Some impairment	Markedly impaired—mistakes unfamiliar for familiar; i.e., nurse is wife	As above

Relations with others	Variable—but most often follows pre-illness pattern	Often clinging; requests help, but can be bizarre and hostile	Usually distant, withdrawn, hostile; can feel omnipotent and megalomanic
Confusion	Variable	Marked	Not usual
Concentration	Variable	Markedly impaired to nonexistent	Variable, but can be quite good
Memory	Recent more impaired than distant	Not measurable	Usually unimpaired
Language	Perseverates, searches for words, repeats, blocks, may be aphasic	Jumbled, mute, confused	Usually unimpaired, but can exhibit mutism, word salad, or neologisms
Awareness of own state	Sometimes—very painfully so	Usually not	Little or no insight
Delusions and hallucinations	Sometimes—but not usually early	Yes—often visual and tactile hallucinations. In delusions, does not feel singled out as sole target	Yes—more often auditory hallucinations; self references in delusions—sees self as sole target
Motor	Sometimes localizing signs, tremor, rigidity	Restless, agitated, tremor, twitches	Most often unimpaired, but can be catatonia waxy, flexibility
Lethargy	Usually not present	Often present intermittently	Not present
Level of consciousness	Usually alert, especially in mild cases	Often intermittently drowsy	Alert

given proper instruction, supervision, and time. Even those "naturals" who seem to have the knack of saying what is useful and therapeutic can learn to make better use of their natural talent.

In addition to classes that teach basic concepts, this kind of skill is best taught when adequate time is given over to various supervised practice sessions. Role-playing exercises, direct observation of the student as he or she is talking and listening to patients, indirect observation of the student through the student's reporting in detail on his interchanges with patients to a specialist in psychotherapy, and videotape exercises with the student alone and in interchanges with other students in role-playing situations are all valuable adjuncts to practicing and mastering the intricacies of listening and talking therapeutically to people who are ill.

The design and purpose of this book does not include a careful exposition of this subject (see Peplau[10,11] and Doona[12] as resources). What follows is a highly selective list of basic considerations. It is a most meager compilation of ideas that can serve both as points of orientation and of departure, as the nurse works to establish an empathic understanding relationship and use it in the patient's best interest.

SUGGESTIONS FOR EFFECTIVE COMMUNICATION

1. Make every effort to talk "with a person" not "to a patient."

2. Start where the patient is. The nurse's attention should be directed to the primary concerns that the patient identifies. If the patient is worried about room temperature, air conditioner noise, the IV drip, visiting privileges, phone calls, husband or wife, or job, that is what the nurse should be willing to listen to, discuss, understand, and use to clarify the psychological issues. One must deal with the patient's agenda in order to build a working relationship.

3. Efforts to establish good communication begin with what the patient knows, understands, and believes about himself and his current problems. A useful question is "What do you know about ________________?" The blank can be filled with "your illness," "your medicine," "your family," "the intensive care unit," etc.

4. Try to see the current situation through the patient's eyes. Attempt to visualize what it is like to be ill, confined to bed, unable to do things for oneself, with restricted contact with family,and just having learned that there is something seriously wrong with you.

5. Listen and look for expressions and feelings. Be aware that people use nonverbal modes as an important part of communicating.

6. Listen for continuity of themes and ideas. Remember that a person may talk indirectly about important concerns by attributing such concerns to others.

7. Do not know too much in advance. Allow yourself to be taught by the patient. Keep yourself open to the patient's unique appraisal of the situation.

8. Accept the patient's expression of feelings even though the feelings may be painful for you to bear.

9. Avoid being reflexly judgmental.

10. Try to respond to patients with statements. Do not use questions as a primary form of communicating.

11. Keep as clear as possible in your mind your own value system and try not to impose it on the patient. When a patient's view of the situation seems "wrong" to you, try to understand what its usefulness is and where it came from. Avoid attempting to argue, cajole, or seduce the patient into changing "wrong" views. Education is a process of sharing, not imposing.

12. Respect the patient's defenses and coping style. You may not like them, but remember that they serve important purposes. Before you attempt to get a patient to give up a defense, consider what the consequences will be and what feelings and behaviors may appear.

13. Speak in plain, serviceable, nontechnical language. Medical jargon and scientific language are often the shield behind which professionals hide in order to avoid talking directly about painful matters.

14. Be honest. Acknowledge your mistakes and misconceptions. Do not be afraid to say "I do not know." Do not promise more than you can deliver.

In-service training programs, both before beginning ICU work and while the nurse is working in an ICU, are the most appropriate places to accomplish the learning and refinement of psychological skills that are directly related to everyday clinical situations. Types of learning exercises and supervision were described above. Seminars, lectures, and reading assignments are also necessary to make the training intellectually satisfying. Many ICU nurses are enrolled in college and university programs and have an opportunity to choose courses that enhance their mastery of the psychological aspects of their work. Where programs are not available, nurses can come together on the basis of common interest and concern to urge their nursing departments, ICU directors, and hospitals to establish them. Genuine need, expressed with conviction and persistence, can be a powerful force to promote the creation of educational programs to help ICU nurses bring better care to their patients.

SUMMARY

Anxiety is the painful affect predominantly associated with ICUs that admit acutely ill, fully conscious, patients. People use a variety of defenses to attempt to modulate and control severe anxiety. Identifying and understanding these defenses becomes an important part of the ICU nurse's professional practice. Ways to increase effective understanding in itself and to be able to communicate the understanding to the patient are among the important anxiety-reducing techniques available to the ICU nurse. In addition, there are other techniques available that involve a systematic reduction of tension-producing stimuli or manipulation of the environment. Depression is seen to some degree in nearly all patients in ICUs, but it is especially prominent in patients with chronic illness and longer stays. It is the predominant painful affect on renal-dialysis, burn, and respiratory ICUs. Understanding that depression may be an almost regular part of the ICU experience for the patient can help the ICU nurse in responding effectively. Understanding that depression often is very closely related to the losses the patient experiences as part of his illness, and empathic communication of this to the patient by the nurse, is one of the most useful ways of helping the patient cope with the depression. Psychoses appear to have become less frequent in ICU populations, although still present, especially with older patients, patients who have had long periods of time on heart-lung machines, and patients who have major metabolic disturbances or trauma that compromise brain functioning.

Learning to talk to and understand people who are sick is a skill that can be taught and that deserves to be an important part of the educational programs offered to ICU nurses.

REFERENCES

1. Hackett TP, Cassem NH, Wishnie HA: The Coronary Care Unit: An Appraisal of Its Psychological Hazards, NEJ Med 279: 1365–1370, 1972

2. Schmale AH Jr: Giving Up as a Final Common Pathway to Changes in Health, Adv Psychosom Med 8: 20–40, 1972

3. Engel GL: A Life Setting Conducive to Illness: The Giving up—Given up Complex, Ann Int Med 69: 293–303, 1968

4. Engel GL: Sudden Death and a Medical Model in Psychiatry, Can Psych Assoc J 15: 527–538, 1970

5. Engel GL: Sudden and Rapid Death During Psychological Stress: Folklore or Folk Wisdom?, Am J Psych 134: 971–982, 1971

6. Dimsdale JE: Emotional Causes of Sudden Death, Am J Psych 134: 1361–1366, 1977

7. Gruen W: Effects of Brief Psychotherapy During Hospitalization Period on Recovery Process in Heart Attacks. J. Consult Clin Psych 43: 223–232, 1975

8. Kline NS, Angst J: Side Effects of Psychotropic Drugs, Psych Ann 5: 442–458, 1975

9. Jefferson JW: A Review of Cardiovascular Effects and Toxicity of Tricyclic Antidepressants, Psychosom Med 37: 160–179, 1975

10. Peplau HE: Interpersonal Relations in Nursing, New York, GP Putnam's Sons, 1952

11. Peplau HE: Basic Principles of Patient Counseling, 2nd ed, Philadelphia, Smith, Kline and French Laboratories, 1964

12. Doona ME: Travelbee's Intervention in Psychiatric Nursing, 2nd ed, Philadelphia, PA Davis Co: 47–260, 1979

CHAPTER 4

The Assessment of the Intensive Care Unit

Nathan M. Simon

Assessment of the unit and the people who staff it are as necessary for optimal operation as is the regular assessment of the patients who enter the unit. Assessment of the unit is best carried out through regular procedures built into the working schedule. Assigning regular times for assessment is a way of emphasizing its value in the day-to-day work of the unit. Regular evaluation done conscientiously and fairly can reduce or prevent forced evaluations that grow out of sudden crises. Crisis-produced evaluations are almost always carried out under great pressure and with great pain to the unit and the individuals involved. The assessment procedure for the unit, when applied correctly, is as nonjudgmental and considerate of individuals as it should be for the patients.

There are several ways in which unit assessment can be carried out, using facilities that are already part of the ICU. For some units, it may be necessary to add a meeting or a conference to supplement the regular administrative functions.

Regular assessment should take place at several levels. The most valuable assessment procedure will provide the opportunities for: (1) self-assessment; (2) assessment *by* leaders of those individuals who work under their leadership; (3) assessment *of* leaders by individuals who work under their leadership; and (4) occasional assessment by people who are not involved in any way with the regular operation of the ICU.

The regular formal opportunities for assessment are: (1) administrative meetings between the head nurse and the unit medical director; (2) meetings between the head nurse and assistant head nurses; (3) shift change report; (4) regular monthly or bimonthly administrative meetings of the nursing staff;

(5) regular evaluations of individuals by the head nurse; and (6) regular meetings of the nursing staff to discuss unit issues someone especially trained to help them with such discussion (See Chapter 15).

The ICU assessment involves examination of the following areas:

UNIT STAFFING

Is it adequate? Is there adequate clerical and other supportive staff? Are staff assignments worked out in an equitable and understandable way? Are there written personnel practices that are known and understood by the staff? Have there been recent changes in the staff, especially in leadership or senior positions? Are there dysfunctional individuals working on the unit; is their dysfunction transient or chronic; and is it being expressed in ways that interfere with unit operation?

ORGANIZATION

Are leader roles clearly defined? Is responsibility clearly delineated? Are there clear policies delineating nurse responsibilities, especially in relationship to physicians and other professionals?

PHYSICAL PLANT

Are the facilities adequate? Is the equipment adequate?

HOSPITAL

Are there good working relationships with other areas of the hospital—administrative, clinical, and supportive? Are there clearly stated procedures involving the ordering and obtaining of services and supplies? Has the hospital provided adequate training programs for new ICU staff?

CLINICAL SIGNS

What is the nature of the patient population? Have there been more extremely difficult cases admitted over a short period of time? Has there been an unusual number of deaths or of crises that have ended unsuccessfully? Are there patients singled out as "crocks" and avoided and disparaged by the nursing staff?

Unit dysfunctioning manifests itself in an almost infinite number of ways. But there are a number of storm warnings that are reliable indicators that difficulties are present and require attention.

There are certain "clinical signs" (to be seen directly by an observer) and "symptoms" (reported by individuals as evidence of distress or dysfunction) that are obvious and understood almost immediately by all the staff involved. In this category are such events as sudden increases in staff absences due to short (one- to three-day) illness, a high rate of staff turnover, difficulty in getting someone to fill in when the unit is suddenly short-staffed, clique formation by small groups of nurses with rigid exclusion and hostility directed to other individuals or other cliques, open, angry interchanges among staff members over issues that are not usually the source of argument, or unusual displays of other types of emotion (crying, depression, euphoria, hysterical laughing, anxiety) by staff members.

Less obvious, but equally meaningful, evidence of unit dysfunction would include the difficulty or inability of the staff to discuss problems openly or directly (this results in problems going undefined until they erupt in crises) and the inability to openly identify mistakes and errors that have occurred. Other less obvious evidence is a marked increase in complaints, often with resentment directed at individuals or institutions outside the unit. This behavior attempts to focus blame and responsibility for all the "trouble" happening on the unit. Scapegoating other nursing units for patients who go "bad," disputes between shifts about responsibilities and work left undone, confusion or blurring of the usual lines of leadership, either by hesitancy in decision-making by leaders or by staff members bypassing leaders in favor of some other authority, are also evidence of unit dysfunction.

The nurses attending a consultation conference began to complain with a good deal of feeling about a conflict arising between evening and night shifts. The evening shift found that they were, with great regularity, leaving work a half hour to an hour late. Part of the problem, the nurses felt, grew out of a situation in which the evening shift had to do vital signs at 10:00 p.m., record them, write nursing notes, and, during the same time, give individual patient reports to the nurses who were coming on duty. The giving of the individual reports kept the evening shift nurses from finishing their work on time. While the situation appeared initially to be primarily a matter of working overtime, it appeared that there were some complicating factors related to it. One factor was that the working schedule was so arranged that the night shift came to work at 11:00 p.m. They were to spend the first 15 minutes getting individual reports and then have a general report from the charge nurse of the evening shift from 11:15 to 11:45. It became an unofficial practice for the night shift to come in a little late, so that the individual report would be bypassed and they would just be on time for the regular nursing report. This meant that, after the nursing report was over, they would then attempt to contact the evening nurse on an individual basis. This would be at a time when the evening shift nurses were finishing up their note writing and preparing to leave the unit. The night shift nurses were not at first enthusiastic about changing anything in the system that would mean giving up the flexibility of having 15 minutes free at the beginning of their working shift. The other issue related to the main matter was that the unit recently had a new head nurse appointed and there was covert testing of the new head nurse's ability to take charge and make decisions.

The new head nurse initiated a series of staff meetings in which the issue was discussed. Gradually a consensus evolved in which nearly all the nurses recognized the problem accurately and understood it. The solution that offered the best resolution was that the night shift nurses would come to work a half-hour earlier at 10:30, that the general nursing report would be given between 10:30 and 11:00, and after that there would be time for the nurses to get individual reports. The new head nurse also had, through the conferences and her own observations, been able to determine that, during the time interval after the early morning nursing report, the night shift nurses were not making maximal use of their time, so that leaving a half-hour earlier would not be compromising the nursing care on the unit at that time of day, which was one of the times when normal shift overlap occurred.

The nursing staff meetings provided adequate opportunity for discussion of the issues. The majority of nurses saw that changing shift times was eventually in everyones' best interests and, after thorough discussion, the head nurse made the decision to change the starting time for the night shift to 10:30. The new system worked effectively. The evening shift were usually able to finish their work on time and there were far fewer complaints about staying after 12:00, which was the normal end of their shift.

The example illustrates the value of a staff meeting system where issues can be discussed, the working out of a logical plan to solve the problem, and the exercise of prompt and effective decision-making by a unit leader.

ICU experience guarantees that some or all of these signs and symptoms of dysfunction will appear eventually. There are cycles in which better and poorer levels of unit functioning alternate. There can be, however, long periods in which a single mode predominates. Prompt recognition of dysfunction offers the opportunity to modulate the severity of its effect. Where the leadership is consistent in demonstrating that assessment of unit functioning is important and that feelings and issues will not be ignored, there will usually be the quickest return to adaptive levels.

Some problems have a chronicity about them that puts an indelible stamp on an ICU. An inadequate number of nurses available for staffing the unit is one of the most frequent of these. Struggles with hospital administration about the lack of understanding of the working situation, personnel policies, and poorly defined leadership roles are other frequent offenders. The head nurse is often especially stressed in that she has allegiance and responsibility to both her staff and her superiors in the hospital administration.

The nurses in an ICU consultation conference regularly criticized the nursing supervisor to whom the ICU head nurse was administratively responsible. They saw her as unsympathetic, dogmatic, and professionally uneducated about ICU nursing practice. They attempted to blame her for chronic staff shortages and other problems. The supervisor actually had little direct contact with the ICU nurses and they saw her as a shadowy, malevolent figure operating at a distance behind the scenes to frustrate their professional efforts to make the ICU operate efficiently. The consultation conference was used by the nurses to vent a good deal of their anger. However, it also helped the nurses to see how, at times, they were displacing anger and frustration from other people or problems. (For example, they had discouraging patient problems plus a unit medical director, whom they liked and felt was supportive but who could not "solve" some of the chronic administrative and clinical problems. Also, they felt that this director did not spend as much time with them as they would have liked him to, but they were not able to be angry with him because of good feelings about him as a person.)

However, the ICU nurses were, in part, accurate about the supervisor who did not make effective contact with unit nurses, was indeed not an expert on ICU nursing practice, and appeared to them more as a representative of the nursing office and administration than as someone who represented vigorously their needs and interests. When a new nursing supervisor was appointed, this complaint disappeared from the conference. The new supervisor had a wealth of experience in ICU practice, related well to both head nurse and staff nurses, and had much valuable professional expertise that she shared with the unit.

This example touches on a number of issues. The easiest one is the limited but signficant value of a conference to sort out problems. However, correctly identifying the problems does not always make it possible to solve them. The more difficult issues touched on are those that develop from the common situation of not having the right person in the right position and the lack of adequate medical leadership. Hospital administrative systems tend to protect themselves, as all organizations do, and even justified criticism is sometimes ignored. One of the hardest types of criticism to deal with in a closeknit organization like a nursing department involves criticism directed at an individual for inadequate or marginal performance. Regular evaluation assessment of all staff members is one way that this problem can be approached. However, even this method cannot always solve an uncomfortable personnel problem that involves borderline or average performance. It often becomes a matter of arguments and criticisms directed against people, which generally are responded to defensively and with the drawing up of sides. However, all good organizations struggle to find the right jobs for people and, when persistent and regular negative reports are made, a mechanism must be available to determine how much of the report actually represents a true evaluation of the person and how much represents the use of the person as a target for dealing with feelings that cannot be easily directed toward other people.

Where administrative problems impair unit efficiency, it may become necessary for nursing staff to become activists. The nursing staff must be willing to doggedly pursue a course in which they bring to the attention of the appropriate people in the hospital—that is, administration, medical staff, and nursing office—the nature of the problems that interfere with their ability to do high-quality professional work.

The tools of individual assessment described for patients are equally applicable to the staff to evaluate the assets and liabilities of individual nurses. Transient episodes of dysfunction are part of everyone's life experience. Leadership in an ICU must be sensitive to the appearance of transient psychological difficulties in order to maintain quality of patient care and also to help staff members resolve these difficulties as quickly as possible. Major psychological difficulties also occur among staff, and sensitivity to them is critical. Oftentimes, transient difficulties are resolved without any special intervention, although an understanding and empathic supervisor or colleague is a great help in hastening the process of resolution. Other times, referral to resources where counseling or therapy skills are available is necessary and will offer the nurse with either transient or major psychological difficulties an opportunity to work through problems.

A nurse, who had worked in a six-bed ICU in another city, took a job in a much larger ICU with a different type of administrative structure. After working on the new unit for some time, she found herself being critical of many of the administrative practices. The head nurse discussed privately with the new nurse her unhappiness about the unit. The new nurse's performance was adequate, and the head nurse wanted to keep the new nurse as a staff member. However, her unhappiness about some of the administrative circumstances related to work continued. In other private discussions, the head nurse talked to the new nurse about the possibility of finding work in a different ICU or, perhaps, in a different hospital, since she was unhappy in her present position and it was not likely that the hospital would change some of the things that she was most unhappy about. The new nurse considered this, discussed it with the head of the nursing department, and was assisted by the hospital in finding a position in another hospital.

This is an example of individual counseling with a staff member over what became an issue that was seen by both parties as not resolvable. Both felt that the things that the new nurse wanted most were not going to be attained by her and, since it was so important to her, it made much more sense for her to agree to leave amicably.

The following example, however, illustrates that such amicable partings are not always possible. A very bright, capable, and aggressive male nurse rather quickly attained unofficial leadership status with the nurses on the shift on which he regularly worked. He was critical of some of the ICU's administrative practices. Some of his complaints were well-justified. The head nurse assigned him to work on a committee with nurses and physicians to make some changes in some of the administrative regulations involving the ICU. The committee work went rather slowly and was negatively affected by a physician on the committee who, at times, was quite insensitive to the contributions that the nurses were making. The nurse became very angry because the work was going so slowly and his frustration and unhappiness increased. He became angry about some other administrative matters and, on one occasion, organized an effort to change a new system devised by the hospital pharmacy for providing patients with medication. Although the nurse said he did not want to be in a position of higher responsibility and did not apply for an assistant head nurse's position when it became open, he was extremely critical of the nurse who *was* appointed. In addition, the nurse also complained about the unit's head nurse, who had been a classmate of his in the critical care course. An effort was made on several occasions to discuss the differences and complaints with the nurse, but this did not seem to resolve the situation. He was transferred to another shift, which made him even more unhappy and which did not in any way decrease his frustration. On several occasions, it was suggested to him that he might be happier working in another unit, and the head nurse offered to be of whatever help she could in either arranging a transfer to another division of the hospital or helping him find work in another hospital. He consistently rejected that alternative. In the consultation conference, he complained about the hopelessness of the situation and, when questioned about it, saw no possible way of resolving the conflicts that he identified except by removal of the head nurse, assistant head nurse, and several other people in hospital administration. Finally, he provoked a situation with the hospital administration that had nothing to do with his nursing practice, but which did result in his resigning from the hospital.

This situation involved a very competent, aggressive, competitive man who appeared to have difficulty in effectively channeling his intelligence and assertiveness. He seemed particularly sensitive to authority figures who were women and appeared to have a good deal of difficulty in accepting a subordinate position to women within the nursing hierarchy. Even though it was recognized fairly early that it would have been in both the nurse's and the unit's best interests for him to find work elsewhere, the nurse himself was unable to free himself from the complexities of the relationship to do that. The head nurse did take an active role in trying to help the nurse resolve the issue, but he was unable to accept suggestions about looking elsewhere, even when the problems were recognized as ones that were not going to be resolvable. He finally precipitated his leaving the unit and the hospital in a way that would make him feel less responsible for what had happened. This example illustrates how personality difficulties can produce considerable stress even in an organization where opportunities are available to attempt to resolve conflicts. It was as if, once this struggle was entered into, its only resolution could be an angry and unhappy one. Even recommendations for counseling outside the system would have not been effective in this case because the nurse did not see himself as in any way at fault and instead would focus only on the frustrations that were engendered in him by an unresponsive administration.

A bright and competent nurse began to quarrel over what appeared to be irrelevant issues with her colleagues, especially with the head nurse. She became estranged from the nurses who had been her closest friends. She called in sick with increasing regularity. Her performance in the ICU became erratic. The head nurse met with her on several occasions and eventually they jointly decided that, because of personal problems in the nurse's life at that time, resignation was the best course. This is an example of a situation in which personal problems begin to intrude in a significant way and are identified by colleagues, and when unit leadership acts to resolve the conflict.

ICU administrators and head nurses who survive for any length of time and are successful at their jobs come to recognize that problems leading to psychological stress among the staff recur cyclically. While the hope always exists that, once the present problem is solved, everyone will "live happily ever after," unfortunately, this is not what actually happens. Periods of high levels of unit functioning are inevitably interrupted by periods of dysfunction. The work that leaders and staff must do to keep the ship afloat is never ending. ICU leaders who believe strongly that, once a problem is solved, it will stay solved, are soon disappointed and find anger, resentment, and despair growing within them.

SUMMARY

Problems regularly developed on even the best ICU can interfere with unit functioning. Administrative mechanisms need to be developed, and implemented fairly and regularly in order to provide avenues for determining the specific nature of the unit and/or the personal problem. Administrative staff and nursing leadership need to demonstrate the importance to the nursing staff of regular evaluation by creating the opportunities for such assessment to be carried out. It is important to recognize that problems need to be solved over and over again. An unrealistic view that an ICU can be problem-free will lead to disillusion.

REFERENCES

1. Di Vincenti M: Administering Nursing Service, Boston, Little Brown, 1972

2. Gannong JM, Gannong WL: Nursing Management, Germantown, Md, Aspen Systems Corp, 1976

3. Haney WV: Communication and Organizational Behavior: Texts and Cases, Chicago, Richard D. Irwin, Inc., 1973

4. Perrow C: Complex Organizations: A Critical Essay, Chicago, Scott Foresman and Co, 1972

5. Stevens BJ: First Line Patient Care Management, Wakefield, Mass., Contemporary Publishing, Inc, 1976

CHAPTER 5

Communication Patterns on the Neonatal Intensive Care Unit: An Analysis of the Effect of Role and Organizational Structure on Communication on the Neonatal Intensive Care Unit

Mary J. Sexton and Misbah Khan

Intensive care units are living evidence of the value society places on the preservation of human life. The use of technology alone is not adequate to insure either the preservation or the quality of life unless effective humane methods of communication are available. This chapter discusses factors influencing interpersonal communication in neonatal intensive care units (NICU), but which are also applicable to other intensive care units (ICU).

IMPORTANCE OF NICU COMMUNICATION

An NICU is unique as a place where communication among staff and patients, parents, and family members of patients is critical not only to patient care but also to the quality of the infant's life after discharge. Facilitation of the attachment or the lack of it between mother and infant may well make the difference between abuse and loving care of the infant, and, in some cases, between life and death for the infant. In NICUs, the highest degree of importance is attached to communication; yet the number of constraints on the flow of communication is greater than in other hospital units. Factors such as: (1) the noncommunicative patient; (2) the volatile medical problem; (3) special and critical family situations; and (4) emotion surrounding the patient are found to some degree in other patient areas of the hospital, but are observed in bold relief in an NICU.

All of these factors may be found at some times in other intensive care units for adult patients, but they are always present in NICUs, without exception. Communication patterns and factors affecting them should, therefore, be more clearly and easily identified in an NICU because of this.

The Noncommunicative Patient

The NICU patient is a newborn infant with no learned communication skills. Except for a few primitive reflex signs and responses, the neonatal patient is unable to contribute direct information about his/her medical condition or feelings other than what can be obtained without any input or cooperation on the part of the patient. The sick neonate in the NICU is like a "comatose" patient, but with little or no history of a normal condition or set of behaviors that will aid in assessing the infant's current status. Unlike most adult patients, the neonate remains relatively passive in the communication process even when "not comatose," although recent findings suggest that the newborn is more capable than previously realized of actively interacting with others.

The Volatile Medical Problem

The medical or technical problems in an NICU are defined on the basis of a smaller range of physiological tolerances. The patient may weigh less than 1,000 grams, a hundredth of the weight of an adult. The physical signs and symptoms are allowed to vary only within a narrow range before departure from a "normal" condition is defined and medical intervention considered urgent. Temperatures vary, for example, over a more extensive range for older and larger babies. Temperatures of one-day-olds with birth weights of less than 1,500 grams have a range of 1.4°F compared with the range of 5.6°F for 13-day-olds weighing over 2,500 grams. For a newborn, a change of plus or minus 3° defines a very small range, and departure from a normal state can be quite sudden. The initial stabilization and subsequent maintenance present a special medical challenge, given the exactness required. As one neonatologist said, "The time and the margin are so tight within which a crisis can develop that sick newborns are far more a challenge in the practice of medicine than sick adults." Accurate and timely communication among staff members caring for and making decisions about the baby assumes tremendous importance under these circumstances.

The Special and Critical Family Interaction

Since the work of Bowlby[1,2] on detachment and separation between children and mothers, a substantial amount of work has been directed toward several fundamental questions relating to the early interaction of the mother and her infant. To retain a simple focus on communication, this chapter predominantly addresses the mother-infant relationship. The promotion of communication between parents and NICU infants acquires significance for those who plan and provide intensive neonatal care, as well as for the mother, family, and infant. One question concerns the optimal period of initiating the process of bonding between a mother and her infant[4]. Closely related to this question of time of contact is the degree of contact. Klaus, et al[5] reported the results of a study showing that mothers who had the usual contacts with their babies, (brief contacts during the first 12 hours followed by 30-minute feeding contacts every four hours), showed fewer attachment behaviors toward their babies a month later than did mothers with more extended contact of 16 additional hours. Klaus' findings of alteration of maternal behaviors are consistent with information about extreme maternal behaviors observed in instances of child abuse. Abused children are known to have higher prematurity rates and are more likely than the general population[6] to have been born by C-section. One interpretation of these facts has been that the early separation of mother from infant puts the mother-infant relationship at higher risk of being negatively affected. The infant's stay in the ICU disrupts the normal pattern of maternal behaviors that assists in the establishment of attachment. There is even more disruption when the mother herself is sick and the baby has been transported to another hospital or another city. We have found it to be not at all uncommon for the mother to have feelings that the baby really belongs to the ICU nursery staff since she has almost no control over the care of the baby. The mother is especially vulnerable to doubting her own mothering skills and capacities with this particular infant. She has little knowledge about her acutely ill or small baby, nor the experience (in most instances) that reassures her about the relationship with this baby. Experienced nursery staff have a vital role in respect to facilitating maternal involvement in the day-to-day care of the infant from the time the baby is born. In addition to providing technical care for the infant, the NICU nursery staff are obligated to keep the mother (and family) informed, involved, and reassured. We believe that the mother who is allowed to exercise her maternal competence in the NICU develops a strong relationship with her baby.

Emotions Surrounding the Newborn

In any ICU, the "work" milieu is stressful. The high staff turnover found in these units has been attributed to the stress and intensity of rapidly changing life and death situations.[7] Society has placed high value on the physical and emotional well-being of the newborn, with the result that the care of the newborn is highly charged with emotion. While controversy surrounds the benefit to society of the life or the improvement of the health of adults at certain ages, no such controversy currently exists about the benefits to society when the infant is the patient (with the exception of controversies around severe incapacitating defects). Society expects the utilization of life-saving medical resources for the sick newborn to be at the highest possible level because there is an assumption of potential for greatness in some area for every newborn. The birth of a baby usually connotes possession and pride in the future. The mother-infant relationship occupies a place of special value in society and is promoted and protected. Promotion and protection of the mother-infant relationship, however, is often complicated by the idiosyncratic responses of a mother (and father) to a specific baby—responses that may either openly or covertly bring the mother into conflict with the societal norms that the NICU staff reflect and represent.

With the four factors just discussed as background, patterns of communication in the NICU will be examined in the following sections. Several types of communication will be discussed—intra-staff, staff-patient, and staff-family communications.

INTRASTAFF COMMUNICATIONS

Nurses and residents spend more time with the baby in the NICU than do any other staff members. The exchange of information between the resident and the nurse, as well as their communication with other staff members in the NICU, is crucial to insure the highest level of care for the infant that the NICU is capable of providing. Yet the organizational structure and the attitudinal milieu within which the staff works are not conducive to ideal communications. The resident physician is in a training position on rotation for a limited period of time, often one or two months. Each incoming resident comes to the NICU with an unpredictable amount of technical knowledge and relatively little experience in its application. The trainee's knowledge and skills are still developing.

Werner, et al[8] addresses the subject of interpersonal skills of pediatric interns. They conclude that graduate medical students need training in relating to patients. The authors state that "House staff training programs, however, rarely include explicit attention to either the interpersonal skills or the general personal adaptation of their interns. As they have been for decades, interns are still thrust into a role for which they are ill-prepared, at times with inadequate supervision and almost always with insufficient emotional support."[8]

The bulk of the technical medical care in the NICU is provided by the resident physician, albeit under the guidance of the neonatologist in charge. A common situation is that the nurse has more experience in both the technical and human aspects of the care of the infant in the NICU. However, the control of the baby's care plan remains within the resident physician's domain. The resident works closely with the NICU nurse who is often more experienced and skilled, but the resident's communication carries more weight and authority with the parents because of the physician's status in society. This is a powerful undercurrent in the clinical setting. The parents value the physician's word despite the physician's inexperience and often his or her inadequacy in communicating effectively. The house staff may be explicitly directed to communicate with parents, but little of the resident's time is devoted to the study, teaching, and mastery of communication skills and involvement with mothers and families. Technical care in the NICU is crucial to the infant's immediate survival; effective communication with parents is crucial for the quality of the infant's long-term survival. The NICU nursing staff and training physicians must balance the attention given to factors relating to the immediate survival with those relating to long-term survival, and must acquire expertise in both areas.

Professional licensure limits staff practice in many instances. Even if the nurse has more experience and skills than the resident physician, the lines of authority remain unchanged. It is the lack of communication, open discussion, and dialogue among staff members about these constraints that tends to contribute to misunderstanding and conflict about staff roles and responsibilities. These misunderstandings and conflicts often remain unexpressed and unresolved. The nurse cannot achieve formal recognition within the hospital organization consonant with her capabilities when these capabilities exceed those of the resident physician.

Similarly, even if the nurse is more competent than the physician and is capable of questioning medical procedures, orders, and practices, this is not formally recognized by a change in her status. An example of the legal position that recognizes the nurse in the role of competent observer is the Darling case of a decade ago, when it was ruled that the nurse is legally responsible for the reporting of any questionable or incompetent procedures. The decision in this case charged both the hospital and the nurse with responsibility for reporting a physician's incompetency. The nurse has been recognized by the legal system as capable of assessing medical procedures and making judgments about their appropriateness. The paradox of great responsibility, but limited authority, status, and power, underlined by this legal position highlights one of the major sources of role conflict and impedance to communication.

Despite evidence that some nurses may be more qualified than some physicians in NICU practice, all nurses remain in a position subordinate to that of all physicians. This situation is contrary to the usual reward systems of organizations. Most organizations reward their employees on the basis of their current expertise and contribution to the functioning of the organization. However, in training hospitals, resident physicians are given status and authority based on their future contributions. This is a common situation for individuals in training roles; they have been selected because of the institution's confidence in their future development. In other professions, the usual arrangement in student training is that the student is closely observed by faculty. The faculty acts as a protector to hide the student's weakness from others while the student is learning. At the same time, the faculty is a corrector of the weaknesses.

This is decidedly different in medical training in a teaching hospital. Here the resident's shortcomings often go unprotected. They are fully visible to the experienced nurse in the subordinate position. Given the responsibility and demand for patient care that are thrust upon the physician from the first day of training in the NICU, it is inevitable that the limits of the resident's capabilities will become known. The resident functions in an open area of observation.

The conflict produced by the incongruity of a person's status and his expertise has been recognized, studied, and documented.[9] This incongruity exists for both the nurse and the resident—the experienced nurse, because her expertise is greater than her status; the resident, because his expertise is less than his status. Even though the nurse of the NICU makes a valid and significant contribution to medical education and training, the nurse is not accorded full recognition. This discrepancy never gets resolved in the formal structure of the intensive care unit. In most organizations, knowledge, information, and skills are converted into power and status. Individuals who have knowledge use it to make decisions and to influence activities in the organization. Some nurses can generate and interpret information and can function at a higher level than can the beginning resident. If the organization were that of a commercial enterprise, the nurse would be a competitor with the resident in the decision-making process. This is formally not permitted in a hospital setting, although, in fact, it actually occurs with some frequency. The lines of authority and rewards of the NICU are like a "caste system" rather than an open, competitive system that rewards according to contribution and ability.[10] The nurse who competes for recognition finds that frustration is regularly encountered when she attempts to exact a position of formal recognition or higher status. One of the reasons for this is the professional status of nursing. According to Katz,[10] the nurse has "no clearly formulated body of knowledge that is recognized and accepted by others."[10] Because of this, she assumes a lower status in the hospital hierarchy.

The nurse who remains in the NICU is probably more comfortable about accepting the subordinate role despite her level of competency; she is able to obtain other satisfaction from her work. It has been empirically established that productivity and satisfaction with a job are not totally dependent on the formal rewards of money and status. In the hospital setting, the nurse's rewards come from the informal system as well as the formal system. In some instances, informal rewards such as peer approval, satisfaction from helping others, and family gratitude are powerful incentives. In the NICU, the formal rewards seem to counterbalance the need for formal role recognition and status.[10]

The nurse usually accepts her position with a minimum of challenge and competition. She is able to accomplish this by using an informal system of communication with the resident. She usually adheres to a series of implicit but well-defined rules with tact and restraint. This approach is the least threatening to her relationship with the resident physician. If, for example, the nurse feels the need to influence a situation and thinks she can do so, she first makes a suggestion to the resident that an alternate way be tried. She doesn't "tell" the resident; she "suggests" that the resident "might wish to stick the baby a little deeper in drawing the blood for the rubella test; it will probably work better."

If the nurse thinks a resident needs a senior physician's help, she first volunteers and asks if the resident would like her to get someone to assist with the problem. If the resident does not respond, she then suggests that the resident might personally call for help, adding that it "often helps in this situation." Only as a last resort does she inform the resident that part of her responsibility is to inform the director of nurseries about all procedures and situations that do not go well. If the resident writes a questionable order, the nurse will ask if it has been approved and, if not, she suggests it should be checked by the senior physician on call. The unwritten rules that the nurse follows in the NICU are steps that allow avoidance of direct confrontation. They allow the resident ample opportunity to accept the nurse's message within the context of the nurse's assisting and helping role rather than an authoritative and superior one. This informal system of communication between the nurse and resident in the NICU requires the nurse's understanding of the delicacy of maintaining the balance between giving a clear message that the resident's performance is inadequate and doing it in a manner that allows the resident to accept it without further damage to professional identity and ego. A head nurse on an NICU summarized succinctly this balance by saying: "It is necessary for the nurse to be assertive but not aggressive."

However, adhering to the communication patterns that attempt to avoid confrontation and, at the same time, exert influence in subtle ways also takes a considerable toll on the nurse. She is, in many instances, forced to tolerate considerable tension while trying to get the message across to the physician who may be not particularly receptive to it. In addition, this type of communication sometimes involves subtle types of dishonesty in the relationship, as well as the need to "swallow one's pride" with some regularity. A considerable price is paid by the nurse for participating in a system that prevents her from directly and openly and honestly exercising her professional expertise and that forces her to play a variety of games in order to protect the patient's best interests. The fact that such systems are supported by the hierarchy structure within hospitals is becoming more recognized and less and less tolerable for nursing practitioners.

Information from the nurse about the competency of the resident gets transmitted and acted upon by the medical director of the nursery. The relationship between the nurse and the permanent physician staff is an important one. The prevailing hierarchical system sometimes provides mechanisms by which conflicts can be resolved. Eventually, the resident on nursery rotation leaves; the nurse stays. The nurse, therefore, may be supported if there is conflict that cannot be handled through the informal channels of communication between resident and nurse. There is a limit to the number of times the nurse can bypass the resident and approach the senior physician with a complaint about the resident. If the nurse constantly uses the direct approach to the senior physician, her judgment and/or ability to get along with the resident are questioned. The potential for conflict is always present in a relationship between the nurse and the resident because of the incongruities between the inexperienced resident's position and the experienced nurse's position relative to their skills. This is a potential for continuing conflict because the resident's rotating system insures a new resident on a periodic basis.

Jack B. Gibbs[13] elaborated a set of characteristics that describe "defensive climates" in organizations. Among other characteristics are those of superiority and control. Superiority and control are quite evident during rounds in an NICU. Nursery rounds are the formal arrangements that permit an exchange of information among all those who have knowledge about the care of the baby in the NICU. While all physicians wish to encourage and benefit from the knowledge the nurse has, the nurse seldom participates fully in giving information and discussing the patient. "Another attribute often associated with full hierarchies is timidity and caution on the part of the subordinates who fear criticism from superiors and thus fear to pass unrelated information up the lines."[9] These perceived threats lead to defensive behaviors, including closed or limited communication.[14]

Of all the staff in the NICU, the nurse spends the most time with the baby. The nurse's observations are invaluable in assessing the baby's status in planning its day-to-day care. The information the nurse has is more likely to be transmitted to the nurse on the next shift than to the physician staff during rounds. The nurse tape records or writes her impressions (depending on the routine in the NICU) in a detailed and complete way. The hesitancy of the nurse to participate in rounds is "expected." A certain amount of intimidation is inevitable during medical rounds for a younger, less experienced nurse. The habit of observation, rather than active participation, during rounds is a long-standing one based on the lack of joint educational experience for nursing and medical students. This behavior is borne out by Haney[14] who noted "By and large, one's communication (as well as his behavior in general) is dominated by the need to protect himself rather than the desire to serve the interests of the organization."[14] The nurse's role in the NICU is inhibited by the formal structure of the NICU.

Shortell[15], based on examination of existing principles of organization, proposed a set of ideal relationships. He states the basic assumption, "That there is a greater need for internal flexibility when the organization is operating in a highly complex, diverse, unstable and uncertain environment than when it is not operating in such an environment."[15] Shortell specifies that a greater flexibility to respond to unpredictable situations results from: (1) low work specifications; (2) decentralized/participative decision making; (3) nonstandardized reward system; and (4) coordination and control without regulation and rules. The life and death situation with the usual emergency, stress, and complexities found in the NICU dictates the need for a high degree of flexibility to achieve maximum communication responsiveness. Yet the formal structure of rewards, authority, and communications of the NICU is not suited to maximum responsiveness. Formal lines inhibit communication between the nurse and the resident because of conflicting status and the visibility of the incoming residents' inexperience. The communications between the nurse and the physician staff during nursery rounds are limited by the formality of the rounds. Personnel flexibility is desirable not only to maximize communication in order to create a harmonious and productive work environment but, most important, to provide the best care for the sick baby in the NICU.

The preceding analysis emphasizes the need for active roles by medical directors, head nurses, and nursing educators to consistantly set examples of appropriate professional behavior. The evils compounded by the rigidity of the hierarchical system and the often nonfunctional organizational styles are less and less tolerable. Shortell's principles can be activated in the NICU setting and can enhance the effectiveness of such units, given the willingness of leaders to take active roles and the presence of appropriate role models.

Another factor that complicates a solution to the situation, however, is the problem of split responsibility. The nurse in most hospitals is in the difficult position of having responsibilities to two separate chains of command. One is a direct nursing chain of command and the second is the medical chain of command. Coe[16] points out most cogently the problems that can grow out of such split allegiances. Some students of the organizational problems feel that developing units with a single integrated chain of command would be one effective way of combating some of the tensions inherent in the "split responsibility" organizational structure.

Communication among NICU nurses is perhaps even more critical to optimal operation of the unit than physician-nurse communication. While it is free of some of the formal organizational liabilities described above, it is subject to its own special stresses. NICU work requires maximum capability for independent action and, at the same time, maximum capability for close teamwork. While assertiveness and independence are rewarded and necessary, exaggeration of these traits, which leads to competition, failure to share, and failure to be responsive to unit needs, is a serious and virtually intolerable handicap. Because of the nature of the work, the usual situation in the NICU is characterized by flexibility and informality among nursing peers who come to respect and depend on their colleagues. The shared stress of their professional life brings much closeness and openness.

Dominance-submission patterns demonstrated in ICU nursing practice, which inhibit free communication and information exchange, are not solely generated by physician-nurse relationships. Nursing in both administrative and clinical areas has its own rather rigid caste system and hierarchy. There are clearly understood sets of "appropriate" behaviors and roles to which nurses are expected to conform in professional contacts with other nurses who have more status and power within the nursing hierarchy. The dominance-submission style, with its marked constraints to easy flow of information from bottom to top of the hierarchy, characterizes interactions among and between nursing administrators, teachers of nursing, nursing supervisors, head nurses, and staff nurses.

Other problems that interfere with the usual open, informal, and free communication among NICU nurses may grow from: (1) overwork; (2) personality differences; (3) poor leadership; and (4) differences over the emotional and ethical issues involved in clinical decisions about the patients.

It is, unfortunately, all too easy to overwork the NICU nurse. Staff shortages are common. The need to work extra shifts is frequent. The nurse is often caught up in a conflict between her sense of professional responsibility and her personal needs. The guilt and anger produced can interfere with optimal communication.

The smallness and intimacy of NICUs make them particularly intolerant of personality differences. Such differences must be recognized early and, if not resolved by discussion and counseling, action must be taken to transfer someone in order to protect the unit from communication breakdowns that affect patient care.

Leaders, either nursing or medical, can become sources of communication problems. Unavailability, authoritarianism, rigidity, indecisiveness, close-mindedness, lack of sensitivity to nursing staff needs, failure to adequately represent nursing staff interests to administration, and the playing of favorites all can significantly block communications and greatly affect unit morale. Providing regular channels and opportunities for discussion of unit problems can serve to deal with recurrent tensions that can appear even on NICUs that function well and are well-led.

Finally, mention must be made of the interference with effective communication that occurs regularly around the tragic and painful situation of the neonate with multiple severe anomalies. Nursing staff can become divided over the extent and vigor of the treatment plan. In addition, the conflicting feelings, including death wishes, are often experienced as unacceptable and unshareable. These feelings can become sources of guilt. Similarly, differences among nurses about the behavior and attitude of family members can become strong enough to significantly reduce or distort communication among nurses. NICU leaders can capitalize on the openness that generally characterizes these units to encourage discussion of these crucial and difficult issues. Nonpunitive acknowledgment of the ambivalences can help restore communication among nursing staff.

STAFF-PATIENT COMMUNICATION

Traditionally, we depend upon the nurse to provide the nurturance and support that all patients need. Maternal behavior and the caring essential to the baby's thriving depend on the mother's early and continuing contact and responsibility for the caring and well-being of the baby. This process is disrupted with the baby's advent into the NICU and is magnified by the infant's health problems. In general, while physicians readily regard emotional health as an important part of the status and well-being of the patient, they look to the nurse and the family to provide that component of care. Similarly, the physician in the NICU attends to the medical needs of the sick baby and relegates the nurturing care to the nurse.

From the point of view of the NICU staff, the baby requires no direct communication regarding its medical condition. It does require direct communication through contact for development. The NICU nurse supplies the care relating to the baby's emotional needs. The mother of the baby may be in another town or, if in the same hospital, may have had complications during delivery that prevent her from being with her baby. Even when a mother is able to visit the baby in an NICU, the newborn requires more specialized care and attention than she or the family can give. The physical touching and expressions of affection that are circumscribed in the adult ICU unit are an expected and essential part of the care of the newborn, if the baby is to thrive physically and emotionally.[17] The rocking chair in the nursery is a recognition of the baby's need to be held, loved, and consoled. This is an instinctive attempt to come as close as possible to "mothering care."

The nursing staff are particularly well-suited to care for the baby because they are responsive to its needs and become attached to it. In our experience, without exception, all NICU nurses are female. Older nurses have children of their own and most of the younger nurses expect to have children. NICU nurses identify closely and easily with the mothering role. The nurse clearly accepts a mothering role and assumes the responsibility of providing care for the emotional development of the baby in addition to routine nursing care on the NICU. The NICU nurse's behavior is similar to the attachment behavior that is seen between a mother and her infant. The nurse talks to the baby, calls the newborn by name, holds the baby, and makes personalized and specific remarks to the baby. The nurse's feelings of attachment and separation are certainly the same as those of the mother even if not of the same intensity. The nurse treats the newborn as a responsive human being and not merely as a patient whose nursing/medical needs are to be met. If the baby dies, the nurse usually feels grief and a sense of loss.

STAFF-FAMILY COMMUNICATIONS

The unborn child has as yet unknown characteristics, even though the baby's existence has been known for the better part of a year. Heightened curiosity and excitement always surround the arrival that has been planned for and anticipated for a long time. The birth of a baby is analogous to the arrival of a mail-order bride. In both cases, the decision to form a relationship for life is made without knowing fully the individual with whom the relationship is established. With the newborn, even less is known than with the bride. The parent accepts responsibility without realizing what the total responsibility is or what characteristics the individual will have. The baby is an object of parental fantasy. The parental image and expectations of what the child will be often mirror what the parents actually are, what they think they are, or what they would like to be. The relationship is established with the child during pregnancy. Toleration of ambiguity and uncertainty is low for most patients, yet ambiguity and uncertainty are inherent in every pregnancy. The birth of the newborn is anticipated as the time of resolution of the ambiguity and uncertainty that clouds the entire period of gestation. The arrival of a baby who is sick, small, and/or handicapped is a *new* stressful event which, even though feared as a possibility throughout pregnancy, has not been emotionally accepted as a reality until the arrival of the baby. What had been hoped for as a happy resolution and outcome of pregnancy is suddenly a sad one with an uncertain outcome. The guilt, disappointment, and fear are superimposed on the stress and anxiety already felt during the pregnancy. The prolonging of that uncertainty when the baby goes into the NICU is superimposed on the accumulated feelings concerning the pregnancy, which culminated in the birth of a baby who is "not normal." The parents feel disappointment and despair when their baby is different and does not fulfill their expectations. The mother has "failed" to bring a perfect, healthy baby into the world.

Not all babies are wanted and welcomed by the mother, and even fewer pregnancies are actually planned or wanted. It is not at all unusual that sometimes during pregnancy the woman is ambivalent about the pregnancy. Parental uncertainty and anxiety about the outcome is present in every pregnancy, as previously stated. We do not address in this chapter the pregnancies and births that continue to be unwanted. Our attention, for the purposes of focusing on the importance of communication, is limited to those babies who are wanted. Women go through tremendous sacrifice to become pregnant, give birth, and provide selfless care for the baby. Making the decision to accept the responsibility of a helpless infant for life is fraught with the mother's fears about her ability to fulfill this momentous undertaking. It is no wonder that, when something goes wrong, she quickly blames herself regardless of how irrational the reasoning is.

The role that either parent may have expected to fulfill is no longer applicable with a sick baby. The care that this baby requires is quite different from that of a full-term, healthy baby. Every individual feels inadequate when faced with the illness of a loved one. With a fragile, tiny, newborn, these feelings of inadequacy are multiplied. The NICU is a strange and forbidding environment for the mother, who is suddenly unsure of being needed or useful and is equally fearful about the survival of her baby. The communications between the nurse and the mother and between the physician and the mother are of vital importance to the outcome of the baby's illness, and needless separation from the mother should be avoided. The nursery physician and the nurse are responsible for keeping the mother informed, for explaining the nature of the problem in understandable terms to the anxious mother (and family), for reassuring the mother, and assisting the mother in the resolution of her personal crisis. The NICU staff must support feelings of competence in the mother and impart to her as soon as possible a sense that she is needed to care for her baby. The nursery physician and nurse must teach the mother and immediate family members how to relate to and communicate with the NICU baby. The nursing staff need to explain in simple terminology the purposes of the monitoring devices and what is being done for the baby. The nursery staff need to encourage the mother to talk with the baby, touch the baby, and, when possible, hold, cuddle, and feed the baby. Without this, the separation between mother and baby may become complete.

Communications between staff and parents and between parents and baby are essential for two purposes: (1) to keep the parents informed about the condition of their baby; and (2) for the staff to acknowledge parental feelings and be supportive of the parents. The baby's changing medical status has to be discussed with the parents, and any questions they may have need to be answered. If the status of the baby changes for the worse, the parents must be immediately informed, especially if the baby's death is imminent.

The mother does not always understand or remember what she is told. Individuals, during crisis interactions, do not function in the same way that they usually function in the absence of a crisis.[18] They demonstrate a more narrow span of attention and comprehension. It is often necessary to repeat the information to the mother on more than one occasion. It is not unusual for the mother, who has been told in the delivery room that her baby will be taken to the NICU, not to remember it. She wonders where her baby is when other babies are brought to their mothers. Sometimes the mother is not told at the earliest opportunity that something is wrong with her baby. She may sense that all is not well. Sometimes she panics. The nurse is usually the first to be aware of the mother's distress. The nurse then either finds the resident physician or any other physician who is available to talk to the mother, or the nurse herself may take the mother to the nursery.

It is not unusual for one of the parents to be told about the NICU's baby's condition in the absence of the other parent. Pueschel and Murphy[19] found that in only 20% of the cases were both parents together when told of the birth of a child with Down's syndrome. The common occurrence is that the mother will be found alone and crying in her room and, when asked, she will say that the doctor has told her about her baby's condition, but she does not understand what was said to her. One experienced nurse has a specific way she uses to handle similar situations. The nurse asks the mother to tell her exactly what the physician said and then asks the mother what part of it she doesn't understand. This way, the nurse assures herself that she is not saying something contrary to what the physician intends the mother to know at this time. The nurse is careful not to impart information that is different from, or in conflict with, what the physician has already stated. Similarly, the resident physician is careful that his/her communications are consistent with those of the private attending physician. The resident tries not to interfere with the parents' relationship with their private physician. The unwritten rule is that there should be no conflicting information given to the parents by the individuals involved in the care of the same patient. Communication becomes guarded and tense under these conditions. Undue care is exercised in communicating with the mother, who is already in a state of anxiety. She is thus apt to be given less information than she needs for understanding and reassurance.

When the family needs additional attention or when communication with the parents or family has been avoided and/or inadequate, the nurse tends to adopt the same strategy with the resident physician (i.e., suggesting, reminding, urging, and then bypassing) as she does with the resident about inadequate patient management and technical skills. As one nurse said, she has to spend an inordinate amount of time reminding the resident physician in as nonthreatening a way as possible to talk to the mother and/or family. It is left to the nurse's initiative to identify the lack of communication and then to seek a solution. As in the case of patient care and use of technical skills, so also with the providing of information about the baby's condition, the nurse sometimes does not have the authority to resolve the problems that she readily identifies. This, again, is a great source of tension. Often the problems clearly would be handled best by the nurse immediately on the spot. However, the organizational structure and role constraints operate to limit the nurse's freedom and to cause her distress in the carrying out of her professional responsibilities. "Game playing," through assuming stereotypical roles, acts, in the long run, as a barrier to free communication. Efforts directed toward maintaining the self-respect and professional integrity of all the professionals involved make it more nearly possible to reach the optimal functioning inherent in the well-organized NICU.

Kupst et al[20] report a study of parents of children with selected cardiac problems. They found that parents were uncomfortable with unclear and vague information. They wanted clear and definite answers and found the wait-and-see stance to be uncomfortable, if not unbearable. They wanted to know the patient's exact condition, as understood by the physician. They preferred to deal with the hard realities of the situation. Most parents want the physician to encourage them to ask questions. These parents felt that the physician did not really want to be asked questions. Unclear communications between physicians and parents of babies on the NICU are similar to the observations made in the Kupst et al study. Many mothers, after seeing their babies, have said, "The baby isn't as bad as I had thought." In cases when the mother does not fully know the baby's characteristics, she fantasizes about the baby. With a sick or handicapped baby, the mother's fantasies may exaggerate her anxieties about the condition of the baby. Some hospitals have made excellent use of photographs of the baby. If the mother cannot see the baby for a period of time and the staff cannot take the baby to her room for a meeting, they will take a photograph of the baby for the mother.

Kupst et al[20] found that parents wanted a written summary of their child's condition, something that they could keep, read, and refer to after the physician leaves. In addition, the parents often ask for an interview with a nonmedical person to explain in layman's terms the details of the medical condition(s). The desire expressed by the parents in the Kupst study to have a clear explanation and some reassurance in language that they can understand is the same desire that a mother is expressing when she is found in her room crying. The nurse helps allay the mother's fears that may manifest themselves if the physician leaves with only a brief or vague explanation, given in an inpersonal manner.

After leaving the hospital, the baby's survival and nurture depend on the skill and loving care provided by the mother. The mother needs to develop feelings of confidence and skill to care for her baby regardless of how uncertain, fearful, or hesitant she may have been initially. The mother must be encouraged by nursery staff to accept her baby, to allow her innate attachment behaviors to emerge. Ten years ago even normal deliveries were managed by babies being placed in nurseries and separated from their mothers and thus deprived of maternal contacts. At that time, only about a third of all U.S. nurseries permitted mothers entry into the nursery and less than half permitted the mothers to touch their babies on the first day of life.[21] Now it is believed that maternal contact with the baby should be initiated and established from the moment of birth onwards. Mothering behavior interactions result, in part, from the baby's responses. A component of reciprocity exists in the dyad. The mother and her infant respond to each other. The mother needs help in initiating bonding with her baby, and the NICU nursing staff need to understand her hesitancy and feelings of inadequacy. The mother can be easily intimidated, offended, or angered by the staff. She can also just as easily be encouraged, pleased, comforted, informed, and reassured.

Some babies may not survive. If the baby dies, the parents need help and comforting during the period of mourning and grief. Smialek[22] describes the reactions of the parents to the sudden infant death. Based on her experience and interactions as a nurse-counselor with approximately 350 parents, she concluded that newly bereaved families need: "(1) Open acceptance of individual grieving reactions, (2) opportunity for vocalizing feelings, (3) clarification of existing misconceptions, (4) allowing the family time alone with their dead infant, (5) provision of a quiet private place to be alone, and (6) an adequate explanation for cause of death."[22] NICU staffs are responding more often in appropriate ways to meet these needs of parents and families.

The death of the newborn is the time when keeping communications open and helpful is most essential, yet it is at this time that it is most likely for the parents to withdraw and cease to communicate with the staff. Parents are especially sensitive to the sincerity and feelings of concern expressed by staff in both verbal and nonverbal messages.

SUMMARY

Interpersonal communication is a key factor in intensive care units that cannot be overlooked or taken for granted. Channels of effective communication among staff, parents, and babies are difficult to establish and maintain. The complex nature of the services, the psychological and developmental limitations of the baby, the intense pace of the activity, the vulnerable state of the parents, and the hierarchical organizational structures of the intensive care units and hospitals with accompanying, often outmoded, role stereotypes all account for difficulties in communication experienced in the NICU. The lines used for warm, interpersonal, and humane communications are as vital to the baby's survival and well-being as are the tubes used for sustaining vital functioning and feeding. Active efforts are required of nurses, physicians, and hospital administrators to develop new and creative ways of overcoming some of the rigidity and limitations of hospital organizational structures and nonfunctional role conceptualizations in order to better facilitate communications and make optimal care of the patient possible.

REFERENCES

1. Bowlby J: Attachment and Loss, Vol 1: Attachment, New York Basic Books, 1969

2. Bowlby J: Attachment and Loss, Vol. 2: Attachment, New York Basic Books, 1973

3. Lamb ME: The development of mother-infant and father-infant attachments in the second year of life. Dev Psychol 13: 637–648, 1977

4. Lourie RS: The first three years of life: An overview of a new frontier of psychiatry, Am J Psych 127: 1457–1463, 1971

5. Klaus MH, Jerauld R, Kreger N, et al.: Maternal attachment: Importance of the first post-partum days, N Engl J Med 286: 460–463, 1972

6. Helfer R: The relationship between lack of bonding and child abuse and neglect. Maternal Attachment and Mothering Disorders: A Round Table, California, Johnson & Johnson, 1974

7. Price ME: Why NICU nurses burn out and how to prevent it. Contemporary OB/GYN 13: 37–46, 1979

8. Werner ER, Adler R, Robinson R, et al.: Attitudes and interpersonal skills during pediatric internship, Ped 63: 491–499, 1979

9. Perrow C: Complex Organizations: A Critical Essay, Chicago, Scott, Foresman and Company, 1972

10. Katz F: The Semi-Professions and Their Organization, New York, The Free Press, 1969

11. Etzioni A: Modern Organizations, Englewood Cliffs, NJ, Prentice-Hall Inc, 1964

12. Eisenson J, Auer J, Irwin J: The Psychology of Communication, New York, Appleton, Century, Crofts, 1963

13. Gibbs JB: Defensive communication, J Communication 11: 142–148, 1961

14. Haney WV: Communication and Organizational Behavior: Text and Cases. Chicago, Richard D. Irwin, Inc, 1973

15. Shortell SM and Brown M: Organizational Research in Hospitals: An Inquiry Book, Chicago, Blue Cross Association, 1976

16. Coe RM: Sociology of Medicine, 2nd ed. New York, McGraw-Hill Book Company, 1978

17. Barnett CR, Leiderman PH, Grobstein R, et al: Neonatal separation: The maternal side of interactional deprivation, Pediatr 45: 197–205, 1970

18. Aguilera D, Messick J: Crisis Intervention: Theory and Methodology, St. Louis, C.V. Mosby Company, 1978

19. Pueschel SM, Murphy A: Assessment of counselling practices at the birth of a child with Down's syndrome, Am J Ment Defic 81: 325–330, 1976

20. Kupst M, et al: Improving physician-parent communication. Some lessons learned from parents concerned about their child's congenital heart defect, Clin Pediatr 15: 27–30, 1976

21. Stevens JH, Jr, Matthews M (eds): Mother-Child/Father-Child Relationships, Washington, D.C., National Association Education for Youth Council, 1978

22. Smialek Z: Observations on immediate reactions of families to sudden infant death, Pediatr 62: 160–165, 1978

CHAPTER 6

Strategies for Tension Reduction for ICU Nurses

Nathan M. Simon

The accurately identified problem offers the opportunity for logically supplied solutions. The preceding chapters have described approaches to problem identification. The chapters that follow will examine in detail specific problems and solutions in a variety of ICUs. As preparation for this, a survey of approaches that have been demonstrated as being useful in reducing tension growing out of nursing practice on ICUs is now in order.

TENSION REDUCTION THROUGH EDUCATION AND SUPERVISED PRACTICE

One of the regular sources of tension in any complex professional practice situation grows from education deficits. There are two components to this source of tension in ICU nurses. The first is the absolute or relative lack of specific knowledge that is necessary for competent nursing practice on the ICU. This problem has been dealt with most successfully in large medical centers and teaching hospitals by critical care courses for nurses that teach the basic sciences (physiology, anatomy, pharmacology, biochemistry) and clinical techniques (reading and interpreting ECGs, identifying arrhythmias, learning to auscult the heart and lungs, operating ventilators and defibrillators) relevant to the ICU. Small hospitals, unfortunately, are not able to mount adequate teaching programs and must either employ nurses already trained in other hospitals or attempt on-the-job training, using a preceptor relationship between experienced and inexperienced nurses.

One reason that patient psychological problems contribute significantly to ICU nurse tension is the relative lack of classroom preparation devoted to these factors compared to the time devoted to other subjects dealt with in critical care courses. In Chapter 3, specific ways to improve preparation and consolidation of interviewing and psychological diagnostic skills are discussed.

The educational process should give the nurse the ability to: (1) understand the complexities of human behavior within the ICU in a practical and theoretical framework that will make possible the development of nursing care plans that include courses of action that deal with the psychological aspects of the patient's illness. This will include recognition of the variety of ways in which people cope with stress and an appreciation of behavior and emotions that goes beyond "labeling" of symptoms to placing behavior, including symptoms, and emotions in the unique context of the individual's life at that moment in time; (2) master the communication skills so that the nurse can share her knowledge, perceptions, and feelings with patients and staff; (3) master the basic skills and understand the appropriate circumstances for their use that can be part of nursing practice to help reduce patient tension and stress and support the patient in the most adaptive coping styles possible in the circumstances of the patient's illness. These skills include reassurance, interpretation, accurate identification of feelings, empathic understanding, behavioral modification techniques (positive reinforcement, shaping), environmental manipulation, and utilizing family dynamics; and (4) utilize the administrative structure of the ICU and hospital to enhance patient care and to resolve administrative and inter-staff problems. In the chapters that follow there will be illustrations of how the mastery or lack of mastery of this part of nursing practice affects nurse and patient on the ICU.

The second component of this situation is related to experience in applying knowledge mastered in the classroom to the patients in the ICU. This type of tension is amenable to some reduction by preceptorship initiation periods to ICU practice and eventually the repetitive successful application in the clinical situation of the knowledge acquired in the classroom (Chapter 9).

Tension reduction is almost always a byproduct of repeated success, which is acknowledged and rewarded appropriately.[1,2] Adequate class preparation and application of new knowledge in supportive, supervised clinical situations enhance the nurse's chances for early success and mastery. Appropriate and effective action is another well-recognized tension reducer. Given relative freedom from emotional factors that override cognitive capacity, the well-prepared, well-educated ICU nurse has available information that allows appropriate action and frees the nurse from the agonizing anxiety of paralysis or the aimless and profitless activity growing out of ignorance.

Regular refresher courses, in-service education programs on new developments in the field, and opportunities to attend special courses and conferences are all additional ways to address the tension that grows out of information deficits. ICU nurses view these activities as high-priority professional needs and are active in initiating them where they are deficient or lacking.

A problem that some ICU nurses may occasionally face is a hostile reluctance on the part of physicians to impart information that competent ICU nurses require to advance their competency as practitioners and to provide the patient with the highest level of professional care. Sometimes this reluctance by physicians may grow out of the physician's experiencing the nurse as an intrusive competitor. ICU nurses should present clearly and assertively their legitimate need for the education and information necessary to carry out their professional responsibilities. Idiosyncratic personality conflicts might make an individual situation an irremedial one with a specific doctor, but clear and precise statements of what needs to be learned, presented with the rationale for the need, will, in most cases, produce the desired result. Even in the face of an initially hostile or reluctant response, the nurse should not be deterred, but should consider other opportunities to make the request and/or clarify the importance of the need. Complete retreat from the problem is usually not in anyone's best interests. However, it is important to separate more general requests for education from specific requirements for education related to a particular patient and that patient's optimal care. Although it is not in the best tradition of collegiality and good professional relations, a threatened physician or busy physician might find more reasons to deny the former type of request. Denial of the latter request is not defensible. Given the limitations of time and personality, sometimes these situations are not resolvable by the two initial parties involved, and the nurse may have to resort to other sources (other physicians and other nurses) for the information she needs. The principle of nurse accessibility to necessary information for carrying out her professional responsibilities is a basic one that must be clarified and defended consistently in assertive and non-hostile ways in all the appropriate forums and by utilizing the available administrative channels. Where discussions among the involved parties are not able to resolve the problem, then conferences with head nurse, nursing office, and medical director may be necessary to resolve the difficulty.

As the popular advertising slogan succinctly puts it, "Getting there is half of the fun." This has direct relevance to the general problem of modulating and controlling tension that the ICU nurse experiences. The very process of instituting a series of actions related to understanding, analyzing, and resolving the problem can yield both immediate and long-range tension reduction. This is true in most cases, whether the problem relates to nurse/patient, nurse/nurse, nurse/doctor, or nurse/administration. As one scrutinizes both one's own feelings and behavior and, for example, the feelings and behavior of a patient who has become a source of stress, opportunities develop to reassess and reevaluate the interaction constantly. The nurse learns new facts about the patient and about him/herself or finds a new framework in which to view facts already known. This can lead to a different understanding of the nurse's own initial responses that contributed to the patient's being identified as a source of stress or tension.

The process of unraveling the specific circumstances and characteristics that make a particular patient a "problem" or a relationship between a nurse and a physician tension-provoking, may, at the same time, appreciably reduce the stress. The process (that is, the ongoing interaction between the parties involved and the self-monitoring engaged in by the nurse) not only makes available new information to be understood in a new light but also allows different types of relationships to evolve. The patient initially rejected may come to be regarded in a more neutral, or even in a more warm and positive, way. The rationalized, superficially compliant acceptance of inappropriate physician behavior because of fear of being disliked can be replaced by more honest, direct reciprocal exchanges. The same benefits of initiating and carrying through the process of evaluation and analysis are possible with problems and tensions arising among the nursing and medical staffs of the ICU or between the ICU staff and administration and can be outgrowths of conferences between two or three staff members or of group meetings of larger numbers of the ICU staff.

STRATEGIES FOR INTER- AND INTRAPERSONAL TENSION REDUCTION

Organizational

ICU organization can promote or impede effective tension reduction among ICU nursing staff.

ICU organization structure is discussed in Chapters 4 and 5. A clearly established administrative structure and chain of command usually decrease ambiguity about responsibilities, which can be a source of stress. A structure that provides opportunities for open communication among all the staff involved on the ICU also maximizes opportunities for tension reduction. While open communication cannot be guaranteed by an organization chart or by a fixed meeting schedule, failure to provide for or encourage regular opportunities for open communication by reserving time for meetings and conferences entails a high risk of increasing ICU nurse tension.

Regular conferences between the head nurse and individual members of the nursing staff are useful tools that can be utilized for tension reduction. Also helpful are regularly scheduled group meetings of nurses with the head nurse to survey unit functioning, exchange information, air grievances, and discuss ways to better deal with unit functioning.

Administrative structure that guarantees participation in appropriate ways in decision-making processes, direct access to directors, head nurses, and others with administrative responsibility, representation on committees and other decision-making and recommendation-making groups that affect unit operation, and a nonpunitive system for dealing with grievances all can promote tension reduction.

Since one regular source of ICU conflict grows from discrepancy in status, power, and recognition between nurses and doctors that are sometimes unfairly related to competency and experience, a vigilant leadership among nurses and doctors in the ICU is needed to set examples in day-to-day behavior and to initiate corrective and instructive action, when necessary, in the

ICU that testifies to the importance of the nurse's professional role and her contribution to unit functioning. A vigorous emphasis acknowledging the nurse's value avoids or decreases the tension that results from the forced assumption of inappropriate submissive roles based on outmoded stereotypes of doctor-nurse relationships. ICU directors and head nurses, who assume an advocate's role for the nursing staff in this delicate area, are acting in a way that will help the ICU nurse appreciably in reducing stress related to problems of professional role and professional status. It will permit the nurse to deal more realistically with professional colleagues with less threat to the nurse's integrity.

Meetings of ICU Nurses With Non-ICU Group Leaders

Two of the chapters (11 and 15) discuss in detail the value of groups led by professionals with group leadership training. These groups tend to focus eventually on more inter- and intrapersonal psychological issues. They make use of a leader from outside the administrative structure of the ICU, who can be somewhat more neutral and objective about the issues discussed, who does not report to the head nurse or nursing office about what is discussed, who can allow the expression of strong feelings in a relatively safe and protective setting, and who can direct the focus of the group to the psychological dynamic issues that relate to nurse and unit tension.

These groups can be led by any one of a number of professionals trained in group dynamics. Nurses with group leadership training, social workers, psychologists, and psychiatrists are all professionals who can be effective leaders of such groups.

Informal Supportive Network Among ICU Nurses

A potent and constantly available source of help in nurse tension reduction is the closeness and sharing that develops among ICU nurses (Chapters 7 and 9). Most nurses find nursing colleagues with whom they are comfortable and with whom they can be open. It is in these more intimate relationships that the successes, triumphs, frustrations, disappointments, anxiety, and tension of ICU nursing practice are shared. Often the process of talking honestly about some strong feelings with someone who is trusted and who understands the situation has a great tension-reducing effect.

Assertive Training and Assertive Action

Effective action is an outstandingly effective resource for tension reduction.[3] Assertive action training permits people to learn to express openly and accurately their views in ways that are clear and understandable, but that involve only minimal hostility. These techniques are teachable. In most large cities with universities and colleges, competent professionals can be found to teach these techniques. There are also several monographs available that are useful as adjuncts or to introduce the beginner to this approach where trainers are not available. They emphasize ways to express ideas and feelings about conflict situations that are honest, clear, and not provocative. The training develops use of language that avoids accusation and that attempts to clarify and identify the speaker's own point of view in nonhostile ways.

Temporary Rotation to Non-ICU Practice

Several authors in this book view the ICU nursing situation as one in which tension is endemic and believe that most nurses in the ICU will experience significant tension with some regularity. One option available for the chronic problem of recurring tension is rotation off the ICU for a period of several weeks to other types of nursing practice. Because of their special educational and clinical experience, ICU nurses can become teachers to nurses whose practice experience has been less specialized. In addition, ICU nurses are well-equipped to work in laboratories that do specialized procedures such as cardiac catheterization or exercise stress tests. The ICU nurse's special education and clinical experience also are valuable assets in preparing to become an instructor in the rehabilitation programs that are frequently offered in hospitals for patients (and families of patients) with acute illnesses, such as myocardial infarction, and chronic illnesses, such as chronic obstructive pulmonary disease, chronic kidney failure, severe arthritis, etc.

Sometimes temporary rotations may necessarily become regular assignments, as the ICU nurse opts to change to a different type of nursing practice, or if unit leadership decides it is in the best interest of the ICU that the nurse be permanently transferred. ICU leaders can also recommend vacations or leaves or can prevent nurses from working extra shifts if a particular nurse is overly stressed.

One other type of rotation available as an aid to tension reduction for ICU nurses is judicious rotation of patient assignment. For a particular nurse, a particular patient may pose problems that, in the short-term management strategy, can best be dealt with by shifting the nursing assignment. Also, there are some patients whose nursing care is so arduous or stressful that daily rotation of assignments may be in the best interests of patient and nursing staff.

Psychotherapy

The combination of pre-existing personality structure with the specific stress of ICU work may combine to make psychotherapy (either individual or group) the option exercised for those nurses who are experiencing tension that leads to significant incapacity in any area of their lives—at work, at home, or intrapersonally. Some nurses will choose this in a completely personal and private fashion. For other nurses, consultation with the head nurse or medical director of the ICU may lead to a recommendation that professional help be sought.

SUMMARY

Two primary methods of tension reduction for the psychological stress of ICU nursing experience are described. The first is educational and focuses on developing programs for adequate preparation prior to beginning and in the initial phase of ICU practice. The second concerns itself with the emotional aspects of ICU work and describes a number of administrative and personal options that are available to help the nurse with tension reduction. These include implementation of administrative procedures that provide open communication, both horizontally and vertically, among ICU staff, regular conferences that evaluate individual and unit performance, participation in the decision-making process, rewarding and recognizing the realities of the nurse's professional role, role modeling by ICU leaders to establish an atmosphere for mutual interdisciplinary respect and trust, temporary or permanent reassignment to other areas of nursing practice, use of professionally-led discussion groups to explore the dynamic aspects of ICU nursing practice, and referral for counseling or psychotherapy.

REFERENCES

1. Beck AT: Cognitive Therapy and the Emotional Disorders, New York, International Universities Press, 1976

2. Skinner BF: Science and Human Behavior, New York, The Free Press, 1953

3. Lange B, Jakubowski P: Responsible Assertive Behavior, Research Press, Champaign, Ill, 1976

CHAPTER 7

The Neonatal Intensive Care Unit

I. David Todres and Patricia A. Rutherford

INTRODUCTION

The nurses working in a neonatal intensive care unit (NICU) constantly experience a variety of stressful situations in their practice of nursing. Many of the challenges and frustrations that these nurses face are common to nurses who work in other intensive care unit settings; several other problems are unique to this particular setting. The NICU is a relatively new branch of specialization in the health care system. Inherent in this evolving field of patient care are several areas that are particularly stressful for the nurse; on the other hand, nurses who work in NICUs reap many rewards and much satisfaction from their investments in the care of critically ill neonates and their families. The following discussion will elaborate on the specific areas that need to be addressed in an attempt to alleviate the situational stresses in the NICU, to enhance the nurses' personal and professional rewards, and to ultimately improve the quality of patient care.

ENVIRONMENT

The neonatal intensive care unit is a unique environment for the care of the newborn infant. It has been designed to provide the most practical and efficient environment for the treatment of the critically ill neonate. While often admirable in achieving dramatic therapeutic results, the unit's design presents a number of problems that need to be addressed. Often the units are at some distance from the referring hospital where the mother has delivered and she is thus "cut off" from the contact she and her infant need to share. The perinatal unit bridges this gap, but this ideal is not always possible. In the unit itself, the infant is constantly bombarded with multiple stimuli. Intense lighting is often needed around the clock for the performance of procedures and the visualization of the sick infant. Sleep patterns are constantly disturbed by procedures; examples—intravenous line placement, endotracheal suctioning, and chest physiotherapy. Noise can be deafening. Noise from monitor alarms, mechanical ventilation, and large collections of personnel in the unit make it difficult for the staff to concentrate on their duties and thus intensify the stress experienced by the nurse. Sophisticated technology is required and is often lifesaving. This equipment may malfunction, however, in which case the nurse experiences intense anxiety until the malfunction can be repaired. She is afraid that this may further compromise the surveillance of the already critically ill infant. On occasion, she may feel extreme stress when an infant is admitted but adequate monitoring equipment has not come through; for example, another pressure transducer that is urgently needed. Often the equipment, including incubators, overhead heating devices, and mechanical ventilators, together with the physicians (particularly at the time of rounds), severely limit the space in the unit, space that the nurse needs to perform her duties in an unobstructed manner. In addition, the parents visiting their infants in the unit are often restricted in their access to their infant because of the limitation of space and the volume of the life-saving technology surrounding their infant. Designers of neonatal intensive care units must be cognizant of these adverse environmental factors, and while designing these units must try to accommodate the family unit in their therapeutic plan. They must also recognize the needs of the personnel working in the NICU, who require adequate space in which to function with the infant, the family, and with each other.

NURSE-INFANT RELATIONSHIP

Nursing the infant in the neonatal ICU poses many problems unique to nursing because of: (1) the nature and severity of the illness; and (2) the fact that the patient is a newborn—a unique individual. The critical nature of the illness is frequently distressing to the nurse[1,2] who sees the infant as a helpless victim of circumstances. The infant may well die, or there is the possibility that survival may be attended by a severe mental and/or physical handicap. The newborn is a frail, helpless being and, not having experienced a previous life, the nurse is left uncertain about that infant's potential future. Frequently, the problems are of an extreme emergency nature, where great skill is demanded and where efforts have to be suddenly diverted from what the nurse is occupied with—thus her concern about leaving one infant if she is caring for more than one infant at that time. The nurse adopts the surrogate mother role; the mother is often absent, having delivered at a peripheral hospital, and her absence may extend to a week or more. If the infant is severely depressed and unresponsive, her emotional nursing-infant interaction is severely thwarted and may be channeled into feelings of anger and resentment towards the infant for failure to respond to its "mother." Often the emotional involvement can become so intense as to possibly jeopardize her nursing evaluation and her caring as part of the team taking care of the infant. She has to take a stand between becoming too emotionally involved and being too distant and uninvolved (i.e., not being a good mother). This is a delicate and difficult balance. Where emotional involvement becomes too intense, the nurse is at risk of developing the now much described burn-out syndrome.[3] Here an emotional situation is reached where the nurse is "forced" to give up her working in the intensive care unit. She quits.

The infant may be seen by a number of consulting services, and conflict between these groups may leave the nurse confused and "caught in the middle"—having no clear idea of the direction of therapy or the correct mode. At times she may report "feelings" that the baby is "not doing well today" or just "doesn't look right"—only to have the house officer dismiss her "findings" on the basis of an examination that reveals no pathophysiological abnormality. She now has to resolve these findings with her own intuition and often this may come from years of experience. Weighed against the relative inexperience of a house officer, she may feel slighted and, if she doesn't have access to more senior staff, has to experience enormous frustration and anger, often towards the house officer. The infant is now "overlooked" while a nurse—house officer struggle ensues.

Nursing the hopeless infant, one who may be catastrophically damaged by intracerebral hemorrhage or who has multiple congenital anomalies that are only compatible with a very short-term life span, may produce extreme anxiety and anger in the nurse. Quite often she feels the medical staff are dealing with a disease challenge—they are treating pathophysiology and are not aware that the infant is a person. The teaching of nurses has always been people- or service-orientated and this conflicts with modern technology, which may keep infants alive who are dehumanized by this process. She may experience guilt over conflicting wishes—feeling it's "better" for the infant to die peacefully, but feeling guilty over thinking this way when it is her duty to treat the infant. Nurses may feel that it is morally wrong to pursue aggressive therapy in certain hopeless situations and are confused with regard to their roles in resuscitation (often being the first person at the bedside when this is required). Unless there is a clear directive from the physicians, and there often is not, the nurse may have ambivalent feelings when she participates in what becomes a "mechanical process." Obviously, in such situations, meetings of nurses and physicians and families may go a long way towards clarifying these moral dilemmas and may provide reasonable decision-making.[4] Dealing with the dying infant can be an enormously stressful happening for the nurse. A sense of failure passes through her mind. What else could I have done? Did I do something wrong that may have contributed to the death of this infant? She has to go through a whole grieving process and, unless she receives the support for this from her nursing and medical colleagues, she may have great difficulty continuing to function in her nursing role with other infants. If the parents have not accepted their infant's dying, the nurse is left to grieve alone.

Reward is important to the nurse and any improvement in the infant gives her a sense of well-being and accomplishment. Infants' conditions change so dramatically that the nurse frequently alters her response 180 degrees from reward and achievement to anger and failure. More favorable outcomes in infants occur to make the overall experience for the nurse a very positive one. This is in contrast to the nurse who works in some adult ICUs where the frustrations may outweigh the positives.

Overwork in the ICU produces fatigue and tension. In this state of mind, accepting another critically ill infant to the unit may produce added stress to the point where there is anger, and this may be vented on the physician responsible for the admission. Guilt may be experienced through these ambivalent feelings of needing to care for the infant and yet not desiring its admission. These feelings are particularly exaggerated if the infant admitted appears to be "hopelessly ill" in the eyes of the nurse. Once the infant has been discharged home or back to the referral hospital, the nurse, while elated with the favorable outcome, may experience concern that things may "go downhill" again—that care may not be optimal. Her concerns are especially great if she is suddenly cut off from further knowledge of what is happening in the home or referral hospital. A continuum of care and feedback is essential and helpful to the nurse. This can be achieved by having patient care conferences with the unit to which the infant will be transferred and follow-up visits and/or contact with the family.

NURSE-FAMILY RELATIONSHIP

The family who has an infant of theirs admitted to a neonatal ICU is suddenly shattered emotionally by the impact of this decision. The normal, healthy infant that was expected has not materialized. A grieving process is underway for the "loss" of this infant and it takes time before the parents accept their critically ill infant as their own. This is compounded by the frequent absence of the mother, who is at the referral hospital.[5] The perinatal center, which to some extent bridges this gap, still takes the infant away from the mother's bedside to an environment which, while efforts are made to "include" the parents, provides a technological arena that is not inviting to the parents who wish to be close to their infant. Recent work on maternal/paternal-infant bonding[6] has stressed the importance of frequent and close intimate contact of parents and infant during the early stages of life. The nurse, understanding this, should encourage their presence whenever possible. She has the important role of supporting the parents through this crisis and seeing the health of the family unit as a priority. The families will often spend many hours with, or in proximity to, their infant, experiencing fatigue and often sacrificing their own needs as well as the needs of other children in the family. On the other hand, there are families who are so distraught as to be unable to confront their critically ill infant and they will stay away. Frequently, the nurse fears the parents' absence will affect the necessary bonding process and may resent the parents for this. She will need to support the parents in this situation and not make them feel inadequate, if bonding is to succeed. In some instances, the parents may feel their infant is going to die and will feel it "better not to get too involved." This is a difficult situation and the parents must be given hope and support when this is appropriate. At times, parents may be unrealistically hopeful, but the nurse must understand that some families need to go through this stage before becoming appropriately realistic.

There appears to be special concern in the bonding with premature infants because of an increased incidence of later child abuse. Thus, special care should be given in the case of the premature infant who is hospitalized for a prolonged period.

The first visit of the parents to their sick infant is a particularly important event and must be tactfully handled to ensure a smooth working relationship and a healthy start to the bonding process. A careful and sensible explanation of the environment and the technology is important, with special focus on the baby and getting the parents to see past the tubes and machines. A healthy participation in normal infant functions should be encouraged, seeing the baby as a whole and participating in its care where appropriate—feeding, bathing, holding, etc. Parents should be encouraged to proceed at the pace with which they are most comfortable. Trying to rush it may result in their reacting in a negative way. Twins may pose a special problem when one of the twins succumbs. One then has to help the family to grieve over the loss of one of the infants and at the same time get them to bond to the sole surviving infant. The nurse should recognize this and provide the needed support, either through her own efforts or those of other services, such as the social service department.

Denial of the critical nature of the infant's illness is frequently expressed by the parents, and the nurse may experience a sense of frustration when trying to get the parents to understand the reality of the situation. Acceptance takes time and the nurse has to appreciate this. Frequently, the family will focus on what the nurse may consider is inappropriate in the light of the child's illness; for example, the parents may inquire of the nurse caring for their infant, critically ill with respiratory distress and on a ventilator, whether the infant gained weight today, and may not focus on what the nurse considers the real issues. One has to understand that the parents, as lay persons, are more familiar with certain criteria of an infant's well-being, (e.g., loss of body weight and elevation of temperature), and that these signs are ones that connote illness and degrees of severity of illness in their infant. Parents are frequently guilt-ridden during the infant's illness, wondering whether there is anything they did that is in some way responsible for the infant's illness; example—the taking of medications. Parents need reassurance here, and frequently the nurse who gets close to the family will identify some of these problems and be able to have the physician answer any relevant questions. The nurse, by virtue of her closeness to the family, is often asked multiple questions relating to the infant's condition—often she is seen as a substitute for the phyisican, who is often seen as "too busy" to stop and discuss things. Also, this might mean taking the physician away from their infant, who may need special attention at that time. Here the nurse needs to be well-informed and to know how well-informed the parents are. This situation often leads to "different explanations" coming from different personnel, and a situation of confusion may develop in the minds of the parents. It is advisable to start off by asking the parents exactly what they have been told and to go on from there; also, to communicate to their nursing colleagues and medical staff what the parents have been told and understand.

PROFESSIONAL INTERPERSONAL RELATIONSHIPS

The interpersonal climate in the neonatal intensive care unit is a major factor that influences the nurse's ability to perform her role in an effective manner. As mentioned previously, the neonatal intensive care unit is a stressful environment that places great demands on the nursing staff, as well as on other personnel. The nature of the work (the severity of illnesses being treated, the constant threat of life or death situations, the pressures due to the immediacy of the work to be done, and the interactions with highly stressed and grieving parents) contributes to the stressful environment in which all professionals must function. In addition to these factors, the professional interpersonal relationships of those working in the neonatal intensive care unit have the potential of creating more stress or of creating a more supportive working atmosphere! The majority of interpersonal interactions in which nurses are involved can be grouped into three categories of communication: Nurse-nurse (i.e., peer interactions), nurse-administration (i.e., interactions with the head nurse, supervisors, and nursing administrators), and nurse-physician (i.e., attending physicians, residents, and interns). An analysis of the professional interpersonal dynamics mentioned here may serve as the first step in alleviating some of the misunderstandings and conflicts that occur; possible solutions to some of the problems identified will also be suggested.

Nurse-Nurse Interactions

Nurses who work in the neonatal intensive care unit require a high degree of competence in delivering specialized nursing care to critically ill neonates, as well as the ability to help families cope with the crisis of having their newborn in intensive care. These nurses generally have a strong sense of identification with the NICU and a sense of belonging to a group with special nursing expertise. In many cases, the common experiences of "burn-out," as well as gratification for the recovery of a critically ill newborn, serve to intensify group ties. Frequent communication and cooperation among the nursing staff is essential to the delivery of optimal nursing care on a 24-hour basis. For a variety of reasons, conflicts among peers in the NICU are a recurrent problem. Oftentimes, disputes arise over the nursing care being delivered. Nurses may be reluctant to share ideas and accept each other's suggestions. Overt conflicts occur at times; but, for the most part, nurses repress conflict with peers, and they may direct their frustrations at other groups, such as supervisors or physicians. This method of coping with peer conflict is oftentimes felt to be safer and less disruptive to the individual who must continue to work closely with her nursing colleagues.

The most common source of conflict among nurses in the NICU is competitiveness. They place a great deal of importance on mastering technical skills (sometimes to the point where the psychosocial aspects of patient care are neglected). New nurses feel insecure in an environment where they are less knowledgeable and are not as skilled as others who have worked in the unit for some time. When a nurse asks too many questions or openly admits fears, she may be seen as incompetent by some of her peers. This attitude tends to reduce the level of trust among staff, who are dependent on each other to fulfill their nursing care responsibilities when they are on "breaks." While many staff nurses are willing to offer assistance to increase a nurse's skills, some competent nurses do nothing to help other nurses increase their level of expertise. Nurses who are threatened by the competitiveness of their co-workers may be reluctant to seek assistance when necessary; others may resent the competition and speak out in anger with those nurses they trust. Neither situation exemplifies an open atmosphere of cooperation and collaboration, which is necessary for each nurse to function more effectively. With the implementation of primary nursing,[7,8] where nurses are accountable for the nursing care given over the 24-hour period, we may see less competitiveness among nurses and more attempts made to bring all nurses in the NICU to a high level of technical competence and nursing expertise.

Most NICUs are small, enclosed areas in which a relatively large number of nursing staff (as well as many others) must work. The procedure of gowning and entering a "sterile" environment tends to cut the nurse off from other colleagues outside the unit, sometimes creating a sense of isolation. Personality and group conflicts may arise "with many strong-willed, independent, aggressive women (generally) working on the same unit."[9] This is not an uncommon dynamic when any group of individuals is working closely together under stressful conditions. Staff meetings with the head nurse as the facilitator for open communications among staff can alleviate some of these conflicts and develop better group consciousness, which will, in turn, enhance the group's effectiveness as a whole.

Nurse-Administration Interactions

A supportive approach to the unique problems of the neonatal intensive care unit is extremely helpful in establishing a nursing unit that is capable of delivering high-quality nursing care. Since the NICU is a highly specialized area of nursing practice, the concerns and problems that these nurses face may not always be appreciated by supervisors and nursing administrators who have not worked in an NICU or who have minimal daily exposure. Nurses may also feel that their supervisor's decisions are not always based on a full understanding and recognition of their needs, and they may resent it when limits are put on their ability to make decisions affecting their unit. If the NICU nurses do not see their supervisors as technically competent, they may not ask for advice or they may attempt to work in a fashion isolated from their superiors. In order for an effective working relationship to be established among staff nurses and nursing administration, open communications must be established. Head nurses, supervisors, and nursing administrators must be willing to listen to the concerns, problems, and frustrations of the NICU nursing staff, as well as listen to their ideas for change and goals for the unit. The most effective changes take place when staff nurses and nursing administration are working together toward common goals for the improvement of nursing practice.

On the other hand, staff nurses who work in the neonatal intensive care unit tend to isolate themselves from other nursing units and are sometimes reluctant to float to other units when needed. This attitude obviously causes conflict with nursing administration. They have become specialized in the area of neonatal and perinatal nursing, and they may lose sight of some of the new trends in general pediatric nursing practice. Nursing administration may want the NICU staff nurse to rotate to other pediatric units in order to gain confidence in other areas, as well as gain valuable experience regarding the growth and development needs of older children. This move on nursing administration's part may be met with resistance for a number of reasons, including a need to stay strongly identified as a member of an "elite" group. Ultimately, the NICU nurse should not see herself as solely a nurse who cares for sick or premature newborns, but rather as a specialist who primarily cares for these infants but who is knowledgeable about the whole spectrum of pediatric nursing care.

Nurse-Physician Interactions

Close teamwork between nurses and physicians is essential to the provision of optimal care for sick neonates and their families. This delivery of highly specialized care requires a high level of competence from both professional groups. Nurses and physicians working closely together in caring for sick neonates have the opportunity to develop a real feeling of "camaraderie," where both professionals frequently share the responsibility of helping critically ill infants through life-threatening crises. Yet, the interactions between physicians and nurses are frequently characterized by disagreements regarding the treatment plan, resistance to accepting each other's suggestions or decisions, hostile or defensive communications, and laying blame on each other for patient setbacks. It is sometimes difficult to ascertain whether these problems arise from actual interactions between members of the two groups, or whether the problems are behaviors resulting from cumulative stresses inherent in caring for critically ill neonates. Both underlying causes of interpersonal conflict between nurses and physicians must be addressed by all involved, in order to maintain effective teamwork and, ultimately, quality patient care. Several characteristic patterns of interaction between nurses and physicians that may result in conflict will be discussed.

Historically, "the predominant behavior pattern between physician and nurse has been dominance by the former and deference by the latter."[10] Physicians have traditionally insisted on maintaining the dominant role in regard to other health care professionals; nurses have generally accepted the subordinate role. The "doctor-nurse game," where the nurse makes suggestions about patient care in a manner so that her contributions seem to be those of the physician, is one example of how physician dominance and nurse passivity have affected their working relationship. Obviously, this pattern of communication is far from optimal collaboration between two interdependent disciplines and has resulted in substantial physician-nurse conflict. In the neonatal intensive care unit, both the physicians and the nurses possess a vast amount of knowledge and information critical to the making of wise decisions regarding patient management and unit functions. Independent decisions made by physicians that affect the *total* patient care situation often result in disagreements, criticism, and resentment among the nursing staff. The attending physician's or resident's acceptance of new admissions, without consideration of the demands on the nursing staff at that time, often results in conflict. Collaboration is essential when decisions are being made that affect the entire unit. Occasionally, resident physicians order treatments or procedures that are not routinely prescribed in the NICU; if nurses request an explanation of the change from routine management, many times the residents resent nurses questioning their authority to make such decisions. Fortunately, this does not occur routinely, since it is important that nurses understand physicians' orders and the rationale behind their decisions in order for them to function competently in their role. When the physician meets with the parents of an infant in the NICU to discuss the infant's condition, prognosis, and possible alternative methods of treatment without involving the primary nurse or another member of the nursing staff, it is important for him/her to communicate what has been discussed. If the nursing staff are not informed about what parents have been told and what their response has been, they cannot provide the necessary support and reassurance in helping families cope with their infant's illness. It is *essential* that the physician and nurse work in "concert" with families whenever major therapeutic decisions are being made. In summary, the physician and nurse must resolve the traditional role relationships of "doctor dominance" and "nurse deference" by working side-by-side in a collaborative effort for the betterment of patient care.

Gradually, nurses are asserting more independence and are moving toward a less passive, more active, role in making their unique contribution to patient care. They are less willing to play the "doctor-nurse game," and they are attempting to convey their ideas and recommendations in an overt fashion. In other words, nurses are becoming more autonomous and are developing a professional identity of their own. This expansion of nursing's role necessitates educating other health care professionals—stressing nursing's unique and overlapping contributions to health care delivery. The nurses in many NICUs are practicing primary nursing, where the primary nurse provides overall direction of the newborn's and family's nursing care. In order to fulfill this role, the nurse extends her personal and professional self to establish a vital nurse-patient relationship, which is essential for the delivery of individualized care to the sick or premature newborn and his/her family. Many physicians may be threatened by this increase in autonomy and authority, where the nurse makes independent decisions that affect the nursing care given throughout the infant's hospitalization. One-to-one communications with physicians should be capitalized upon as opportunities for nurses to explain their functions and goals and to clear up misunderstandings that nurses are seeking to take power away from physicians. An enlightened physician, Barbara Bates, has remarked that nursing only "wants access to the patient and sufficient control over the nurse-patient encounter to deliver its own unique product, full nursing care."

In the neonatal intensive care unit, teamwork is essential to achieve optimal utilization of each discipline's expertise in treating sick or premature neonates. There is an intense need for collaboration among physicians, nurses, social workers, and other professionals. This discussion will focus primarily on the physician's and nurse's roles as team members. The traditional roles of nurses and physicians are frequently violated in actual practice in the NICU. There are several reasons for this: (1) Neonatology is a highly specialized field of medical and nursing practice; (2) there is a constant influx of new personnel (primarily interns and residents training for from four to eight weeks in the NICU);[11] and (3) the immediacy of emergencies and crisis situations necessitates that the physicians and nurses often perform the same, and, at times, each other's tasks. "The consequent lack of clearly understood role expectations and task definitions leads to ambiguity, confusion, and sometimes strife." One perennial source of difficulty is a result of the frequent change in intern or resident coverage of the NICU; they are generally less knowledgeable about the general care of neonates, techniques, equipment, and routine procedures than are their nursing colleagues. Although these residents are supervised by the attending physician and senior residents, they are frequently dependent on the nursing staff for guidance and suggestions regarding the physician's management of patient care. This situation frequently leads to role conflict. Once the resident becomes more knowledgeable, he/she becomes less dependent on the nursing staff. Another area of conflict that frequently occurs is the "policing" of one another's activities and performance. Such conflicts can only be resolved through open communication between the unit directors and nursing leadership staff in order to clearly define the roles of nurses and physicians, as well as the delegation of authority to make decisions and resolve problems. The interdependent nature of medicine and nursing necessitates this mutual sorting out of responsibilities so that physician-nurse conflicts will be lessened. Once the roles and responsibilities are more clearly defined and communicated to those working in the NICU, hopefully, collaboration will take the place of competition and more effective teamwork will be established.

When an infant is critically ill, all who are close to him go through a profound emotional experience. The neonatal intensive care unit is a crisis-laden environment that places a great deal of pressure and stress on those who work there. The stresses within the environment, the patient-related concerns and frustrations, and the emotional toll of helping stressed and grieving parents are common to both nurses and physicians who work in the NICU. The cumulation of these stresses often creates an atmosphere of strife, which can adversely affect the relationships of those working together. On the other hand, open communication between nurses and physicians can enhance their working relationship, creating an atmosphere of mutual support. This can be accomplished through informal discussion, one-to-one communication, and group meetings that give members the opportunity to vent feelings, anxieties, and concerns.[12]

SUMMARY

The neonatal ICU has improved the prognosis for the critically ill newborn and particularly the low-birth-weight infant. This unique environment has brought together the sophistication of modern medical technology and the skills of specially trained health care personnel—physicians, nurses, laboratory technicians, respiratory therapists, social workers, and others. This complex team working in an intense "mechanical" environment must develop a system of harmony if it is to succeed in its aim; namely, the welfare of the sick infant and its family. "In a setting of high ego involvement by the staff, saving lives is not a small matter."[12] The nurse, as a vital member of this team, has to develop technical skills as well as human relationship qualities that will allow her to carry out her responsibilities in an optimal manner. The nurse's work in the NICU produces great rewards, but also frequently produces unique stresses and strains that have to be confronted and worked through. As Cassem et al so aptly stated, "Paradoxically, the source of the greatest stress and of the greatest satisfaction is the same: Caring for desperately ill patients."[13]

For the nurse to fulfill her role in the NICU, she needs to recognize her sense of worth and value in the care of the sick neonate; to understand her feelings at times when she "loses the battle" to save the life of the infant; to recognize that she is a member of a team and needs to share a mutual goal with each member of the team; and to improve the health and future happiness of newborn infants and their families.

REFERENCES

1. Jacobson SP: Stressful situations for neonatal intensive care nurses. Maternal Child Nursing 3: 144–152, 1978

2. Surveyer JA: The emotional toll on nurses who care for comatose children. Maternal Child Nursing 1: 243–248, 1976

3. Shubin S: Burnout: The professional hazard you face in nursing. Nursing 78: 22–27, 1978

4. Benfield DG, Leib SA, Vollman JH: Grief response of parents to neonatal death and parent participation in deciding care. Pediatrics 62: 171–177, 1978

5. Benfield DG, Leib SA, Reuter J: Grief response of parents after referral of the critically ill newborn to a regional center. N Engl J Med 294: 975–978, 1976

6. Klaus MH, Kennell JH: Maternal-infant bonding, St. Louis, C.V. Mosby Company, 1976

7. Marram D, Schlegel W, Bevis EO: Primary nursing: A model for individualized care, St. Louis, C.V. Mosby Company, 1974

8. Spoth J: Primary nursing: The agony and the ecstasy. Nursing Clinics of N Amer 12: 221–234, 1977

9. Bilodeau CB: The nurse and her reactions to critical care nursing. Heart and Lung 2: 358–363, 1973

10. Kalisch BJ, Kalisch PA: An analysis of the sources of physician-nurse conflict. J Nurs Admin 51–57, 1977

11. Todres ID, Howell MC, Shannon DC: Physicians' reactions to training in a pediatric intensive care unit. Pediatrics 53: 375–383, 1974

12. Rosini LA, Howell MC, Todres ID: Group meetings in a pediatric intensive care unit. Pediatrics 53: 371–374, 1974

13. Cassem NH, Nelson K, Rich RR: The nurse in the coronary care unit. *In* Gentry WD, Williams RB (eds): Psychological aspects of MI and coronary care, St. Louis, C.V. Mosby Company, 1975

CHAPTER 8

Psychological Aspects of Pediatric Intensive Care Nursing

George Albertus, Francine Guldner, and Harriet Pollard

INTRODUCTION

In recent years the medical literature has come to recognize that the quality of patient treatment in intensive care may depend as much upon the psychological well-being of the nursing staff as on their technical competence.[1,2] The stresses on nurses working with patients whose lives are at stake can be tremendous. Coping successfully with these stresses is crucial to the care-giving capability of the nurse and ultimately may relate to the outcome of the patient.

The reduction of stress begins with accurate identification of issues that are stressful. This, in itself, can reduce confusion and stress by determining where attention needs to be focused and what elements need to be changed. From more realistic assessment comes the understanding needed as a guide to action.

This chapter discusses the sources of stress identified by the authors in their pediatric intensive care units. The nursing experiences presented are by no means all limited to a pediatric ICU. Many are unique to the care of children, while many more are common to a variety of ICU and hospital environments. The clinical setting has been described as a whole in the hope of providing insight into the improved management of similar stresses wherever they may be found.

ENVIRONMENT

St. Louis Children's Hospital is a 182-bed pediatric hospital that includes four intensive care units. The large neonatal ICU is staffed separately from the three units to be considered here, which share 34 staff RNs, three clinical nurses, two LPNs, and one patient care manager (head nurse). All but 14 staff nurses are full-time.

The smallest of the ICUs specializes in cardiac patients, and all children who have open heart surgery go there postoperatively. The unit was planned for three patients, but it often holds four in its 420 square feet. A five-bed ICU of 500 square feet cares for patients with neurological and neurosurgical problems. It also receives overflow from the general ICU which, at 715 square feet, is the largest of the three units. The general ICU is also the busiest of the units and serves the greatest variety of patients, including general surgery, trauma, burn, and infectious disease. One of its five beds is in a glass-doored isolation room.

Located in the midst of separate patient divisions at Children's Hospital, the intensive care units show little sign of the intense realities that are played out within. Like many of their patients, the units are small and have been fitted into space not originally meant for their use. They serve their functions well, however, and only space and some convenience will be gained in new facilities.

A sign hangs outside each unit, thanking visitors for cooperating with the following restrictions: only two visitors at a time per patient; no visiting during nursing report, doctor's rounds, and emergencies; visits may be restricted when the unit is busy. If the door is closed for one of these reasons, another sign may suggest a later visit. A lounge for parents and visitors is available, though not adjacent to the unit, and each lounge is equipped with phone, television, and sleeping accommodations.

Inside a unit, the walls are covered with supply shelves, lights, connections, and monitors. Wall space too high to be usable displays a few posters with messages on caring: "Love is taking care of somebody." "No act of kindness, no matter how small, is ever wasted." Supplies and equipment that the shelves cannot accommodate are left on the floor, to be moved as space and use require. All of the units have outside windows, but they do little to change the office-like brightness of constantly shining multiple fluorescent lights.

Without patients, the units are quiet and spacious with clean floors and echoes. With patients, each unit is itself again, a clutter of equipment and beds, personnel, and relatives who somehow find their own space.

To the outsider entering a unit, there seems to be a barrage of assaults on both the senses and the emotions. From every quarter of the room come mechanical cries for attention, as buzzes, beeps, and whooshes compete with steady red, flashing yellow, and bouncing blue lights. Wires, tubes, switches, and gadgets seem to be everywhere, but particularly coming out of the patients themselves.

Confined to their beds on their backs, the more seriously ill infants and children seem to have bodies defiled by every possible combination of connection and invasion, their faces hardly recognizable beneath the mask of tape holding tubes in place, their extremities restrained and conforming to the shape of boards that protect precious IVs. Blood, stool, urine, and stomach drainage often stain the bed linen, which may or may not also cover the patient's body, as his care, rather than modesty, dictates.

For the uninitiated, this scene evokes surprise, repulsion, sadness, and curiosity, for it is a setting where children are not really themselves, but prisoners of the hospital and of their illnesses. They do not look the way children usually look; they do not act the way children usually act. Their communication, in whatever form, is basic: something to eat or drink; a bedpan or a dry diaper; it hurts here, please make it stop. Their manner is subdued and inhibited as their bodies struggle to regain health and throw off pain and discomfort.

Those patients with less severe problems or who are well along in their recovery may be awake and alert, sitting up, playing, or watching TV. For the nursing staff, these patients are a pleasant change of pace. The joy of the young can be found in an ICU, but its appearances are, on the whole, fleeting and few. By the time a child feels like resuming normal activity, he has probably been transferred from the intensive care unit that he no longer needs.

In time, the sharp edges of the ICU are softened by familiarity and confidence in one's abilities, yet the special reality of intensive care is an unrelenting one for the nurse. Unless the unit is especially slow or staffing especially good, the only relief, short of going home, may be quick trips for food or to the toilet. If staff lounges were available for temporary retreat, the nurse would have difficulty getting away to use them.

Numerous alarms, machines, phone calls, doctors, parents, and visitors may make more demands on the nurse than do the patients, who are often unable even to express their needs. The inexperienced house officer may be unsure of what *should* be done for the patient; the family is anxious about what *can* be done; the patients are upset by what *is* done; and it is around the "doing" of the nurse that all of these feelings revolve.

Though there is the potential for many nursing actions to be life-saving, they may also be life-threatening if the proper decision is not made at one of the crucial times, which can occur at any moment. Death and dying are constant shadows in the ICU. They demand a certain hopefulness for the potential of the sick child, in the face of frequent demonstrations that, for some, this potential will never be realized. With experience, the nurse may recognize death long before it arrives, making the loss of life all the harder, as it slips away while care must be provided as though it were returning.

Most of the children, though, begin to recover, are transferred out, and eventually go home. The spaces they leave are never empty long, for in ICU the only real constants are sickness and the struggle to overcome it. Patients and parents, interns, residents, and nurses spend their time and make way for others in a never-ending procession of those with special abilities striving to meet the demands of those with very special needs.

STAFFING

Growing out of the demands of its patients, the workload of the ICU may remain constant for long periods or it may change in a matter of minutes. Therefore, staffing is a perpetual problem. The greatest activity occurs during the day shift, when most physicians' rounds are made, baths are given, and beds, tubings, and fluids are changed. There is also an abundance of support personnel, including respiratory care, laboratories, transporting, housekeeping, and central supply. On the evening shift, there is less commotion, but patients with longer and more complicated surgeries often return then and more relatives are able to visit.

The night shift is likely to be the quietest, with routine care and preparation for morning diagnostic tests, but it can also be the most eventful, since there is less staff, and some of the most acutely ill children arrive from outlying areas during the night. Often the night nurse is responsible not only for drawing blood work, but for transporting it to the lab. When housekeeping is not available, she may have to clean a unit in order to receive a new patient, who may also have an extended wait for equipment or supplies. Respiratory care and treatments may be difficult to obtain because of a shortage of therapists at night. These problems, along with added secretarial duties, place an extra burden on the night nurse, who is probably working with less than ideal staffing.

The night shift is least preferred by the staff, probably because it is the most disruptive to a normal personal life. Consequently, new staff members usually work at least some nights, then request transfer to more favorable hours. This again leaves a night position to be filled by the next new person.

Vacations, absences, and illnesses create holes in the ICU schedule that must be filled by the remaining staff. This problem is worse on the night shift, holidays, and weekends, which are already minimally staffed. Few, if any, of the remaining staff are willing to sacrifice precious time off or to rearrange their bedtime to stay up all night to work.

Although ICU nurses may be called to work on regular patient divisions from time to time, the work in intensive care is sufficiently specialized and demanding that nurses from outside the units cannot fairly be called in when extra help is needed. Therefore, all replacements must come from within the ICU staff. The result can be the frequent experience of calls during the nurse's day off to come in to work.

If no one can be found, those working may need to come in early or stay late, perhaps working two consecutive shifts—a "double"—simply because there is too much to do and there are too few to do it. This creates a persistent morale problem if the overload continues, as the nurse desires simply to finish her shift and seek relief outside the hospital setting, unable to do justice to either her personal or professional life.

THE ROUTINE

The closeness of the walls and all that they must contain contribute to the intensity of the ICU nursing, but it is the basic routine of patient care that holds the nurse within this environment and occupies her attention so fully during the time on duty. It is a time of complete responsibility. In the ICUs there are no aides, no nurses specially designated to take charge, give medicines, or lead the nursing "team." For each child, that team is one nurse.

Each gives her patient's medicines, carries out all of his orders, and deals with his parents and relatives. A nurse may have more than one patient, but, for each of them, that nurse is the provider of the care the child needs and has been ordered to receive.

Routine in the ICU is heavily structured, both for the sake of providing consistent, continuing care, and for regular assessment of the patient's condition. The basic unit of time is the hour, with the great majority of medicines, vital signs, fluid readings, and special procedures scheduled to fall on the hour. This presents a secure routine for the nurse to fall into, with definite obligations to be fulfilled at definite times. But it also can be very frustrating when the unexpected obligation conflicts with the regular duty, as in an emergency, or with the child who manages to pull out his feeding tube at the same time IV checks, antibiotics, blood work, and complete vital signs are due.

For the acutely ill or postoperative child who is on a respirator with chest tubes, arterial lines, and multiple IVs and medications, the hourly duties may be so complicated and numerous that by the time one set is finished it is already time to begin the next. Two or three less serious but demanding patients can easily produce the same unending race with the clock; a race the nurse knows she is destined to lose before it is begun.

Conceivably, this leaves no time for talking to parents, eating lunch, or helping another nurse with a task requiring four hands. Yet these, too, must be accommodated in a work schedule that is already lapping itself on the hour. The consequence can be overtime at the shift's end, as the nurse gives up personal time to catch up on work that her other work didn't allow her time to get finished. More often, it means accomplishing the essentials first, without ever getting to such niceties as the nurse's uninterrupted meal or the patient's care plan, which are deserved, but not demanded.

The repetitive time conflict in ICU demands that the nurse not only adjust work speed to the amount of work to be done, but be able to make assessments quickly and determine priorities. Once gathered, the various pieces of information on each patient must be charted and acted upon as necessary. The conscientious nurse may be left wondering what was missed in the rush of duty and data—"Was this child trying to tell me something that I was too busy to hear?"

In an arrest situation, where 20 persons are trying to occupy space meant for five and each of several doctors is requesting something different immediately, it is inevitable that some patient care will have to be postponed or will go undone. The arrest itself, and keeping the child's parents informed, rate high priorities, while a low potassium, an infiltrated IV, and a wet diaper elsewhere in the unit may have to wait until the crisis is past. Determining what has to be done and doing it as efficiently as possible requires of the ICU nurse a decisive mind and the ability to separate the crucial from the merely significant, the necessary from that which can wait.

PATIENT CARE

In the everyday care situation, objectives are more general and less explicit than in the crisis of an emergency. For the nurse, this means it is more likely that there will be time to give the care that is needed, but it also allows a great deal of freedom in deciding how, and to whom, this care is to go.

Those children whose care is most attractive to the nurse, often regardless of their condition or the amount of work involved, will receive most of that nurse's attention. Those children whose care is unattractive to the nurse will receive the least of her attention. Doctors' orders and hospital routine guarantee each patient certain measures for the recovery of health, but it depends on the nurse applying those measures as to how carefully they are accomplished and how much personal attention accompanies them.

Patient care attractiveness can be very different for different nurses, and does not necessarily include the cherubic features of the cute and smiling child. Physical attractiveness may be initially appealing, but over an eight-hour period it is easily overshadowed by demands the nurse considers excessive from the patient or his family. An angelic countenance is little compensation for returning to the bedside every few minutes to do and redo minor tasks or to answer endlessly repetitive questions from anxious parents. Even the infant or newborn soon demonstrates his personality to those caring for him, and the cute, but wiggly, irritable baby who shows a temper is unlikely to gain nursing favor.

Similarly, physical deformity may not be at all unattractive when accompanied by a pleasing and agreeable personality. Four-year-old Marcia, who had a monstrous upper neck mass, was a favorite of hospital employees for her loving behavior and unique sense of humor, which quickly removed any sense of ugliness from her grossly distorted face.

The chronically ill child who manages to maintain a certain sense of identity and independence of spirit in spite of his affliction often evokes great empathy and much affection from nurses. Daniel had been admitted six times in his five years for complications of cystic fibrosis and required frequent suctioning and position changes. Though he required much care, he did not demand attention, and gave the feeling that he was doing his part in the never-ending struggle into which he was born. As a result, his care was attractive to most nurses, and he received a good deal of extra personal attention.

While Daniel was an appealing patient, he required a lot of energy, both emotional and physical. Those who cared for him on a regular basis sometimes found themselves needing a break from the demands of his care. If the nurse remained in the unit but took another patient, she felt she was expected to continue working with Daniel, yet at the same time she needed the chance to recover the energies depleted by his care.

A patient's appeal to the nurse is influenced not only by the demands of his care, but by the nurse's perception of her ability to meet those demands. The same factors of complicated care, a particularly critical illness, and the need to work closely with physicians that make a patient with Reye's syndrome challenging for some nurses can just as easily make the care of that patient unattractive to the inexperienced or less confident nurse. The fear of not knowing what to do in an emergency or of being embarrassed by making a mistake is reason enough to avoid working with such a patient, regardless of other patient or family characteristics.

The amount of effort a patient's condition requires can also make his care unattractive for the nurse who is tired or less ambitious. Generally, the more tubes, medicines, and complications a patient has, the more work he will require. Most nurses consider a patient on isolation to be an extra burden, as the gloves, gown, and mask take time to put on and take off each time the patient is approached and can be hot and restrictive to work in. Given a choice, it is easier to take a patient who is less sick and less involved, though it may be ultimately less satisfying for the nurse, as well as more straining on her relations with co-workers, if she always avoids the more difficult patients.

In the Children's Hospital ICUs, no patient assignments are made, and it is up to the nurses in each unit to decide who will care for which patients. For the nurse receiving duties she considers unattractive, this can mean a full shift with a child whose demands outweigh the satisfactions she receives. This is an energy-draining experience and is impossible to maintain day after day. To some nurses, burned children fit into this category, with their restrictive isolation procedures, the need to inflict pain in involved dressing changes, parents experiencing deep guilt, and a long, slow, healing process. There must be an opportunity for relief from those situations that deplete the nurse's energies without replacing them or the patient's care will take place at the expense of the nurse's own well-being.

RETREAT

The ICU environment is not only physically small, but restrictive, as the nurse must be in the room for nearly all of her time on duty. During times of stress, whether major crisis or minor emergency, flight is not an acceptable alternative. This constant exposure to patients, parents, and doctors, without retreat, provides the impetus for the nurse to develop other means of withdrawing from uncomfortable situations.

A large number of pediatric patients are too young to talk or to relate personally to those caring for them. Apart from basic care, the infant who is unattractive to the nurse can simply be left alone, with no need for explanation or pretense. The unconscious or acutely ill child can be similarly treated as long as the nurse's conscience does not protest too loudly.

When the patient who is considered unattractive can communicate and would know when he is being avoided, the "busy work" of intensive care routine provides an easy refuge for the nurse. There is always some little thing to be done elsewhere in the room, whether it is paperwork, medicines, regulating IVs, or attending to another patient. Even when the child is aware that he is being avoided, it is most unlikely that he would confront the nurse about it.

The "something else I've got to do" retreat may also be used with parents and other relatives. A short, uninformative answer and a return to other duties is one means of avoiding contacts that might involve the strong emotions and unusual behavior of family members who are having difficulty coping with the child's illness. Intensive care does mean many duties that preempt prolonged dealings with a child's family. Orders for care are written for patients, not their families, and the easy way to avoid this unwritten obligation is to turn to the definite tasks of patient care.

The distancing of patient or relative by refusing personal, sympathetic interaction is, however, directly contrary to the nurse's role of aiding the child's return to health and his position in the family. It is quite possible to provide the reassurance and information needed even when time is limited. A smile, a meeting arranged with a doctor to answer questions, a chair at the patient's bedside, or a quick trip to the parents' lounge to keep them informed take little extra effort on the part of the nurse, but can make the difference between caring only for the child or caring for the child and his family.

PAIN

Habituation of some degree is unavoidable for the ICU nurse, who must always work in the shadow of a potential crisis. Emotional responses become dulled by the frequency with which they are elicited and the recurrent need to push them aside in favor of more pressing matters. It is not only necessity, but denial, that allows the nurse to eat a meal in the unit amidst scenes that would cause the average person to lose all interest in eating. In order to remain in intensive care, the nurse must learn not to get too emotionally involved in what goes on there and, in the process, adopt some mechanisms that serve to dehumanize both patient and self.

Many nursing actions are distressful to the pediatric patient, who seldom takes kindly to being probed with electronic thermometers, cajoled into consuming medicine when the smell lies about its taste, or having to stay immobilized in bed because everything that moved was tied down. Perhaps most distressful to the nurse are those tasks that require inflicting pain on the children under her care.

In a direct conflict of loyalties, the nurse must carry out the orders and routine of the medical system of which she is an integral part, while being charged with the utmost consideration for the well-being of her patients. Where pain is concerned, fidelity to both is not possible, and in the end it is the child who is betrayed and the nurse who must cope with the betrayal.

Starting IVs, giving injections, and drawing blood all require the painful, and often repetitive, invasion of the child's body with needles by the nurse. Endotracheal suctioning, burn dressings, and chest tube stripping can also mean significant pain for the child. As an accomplice, the nurse must also share with the physician the hurt inflicted during venous cutdowns, thoracotomies, and lumbar punctures, a hurt often without benefit of anesthetics, which might interfere with the procedure and which are easier to do without when the patient is too young to verbalize his pain.

It is the position of the nurse to be comforter, surrogate parent, and caretaker to the child, gaining his confidence as someone who can be counted on for support in a strange world where he does not feel like himself and does not know what to do about it. Then, with the same quiet words and careful hands he had come to trust, she brings him terrible pain, for which "You're all right" and "It's almost over" are no help at all. The child is left, hurting and betrayed, while the nurse must reconcile the desirability of restoring health to the child with the pain of methods that her training has taught her are necessary to achieve it.

Fortunately, children are quick to forget and forgive, and their fear is often impersonally expressed—the needles receive the distrust rather than the person bringing them. Yet the need to willfully cause a child pain is a difficult dilemma for the concerned nurse.

The simplest mechanism to assume in dealing with the hurt the nurse must cause is isolation, wherein an action, such as drawing blood, is given the same matter-of-fact treatment as filling an IV or washing one's hands. Both the feelings of the child and of the nurse are ignored, as the painful deed is mechanically carried to completion.

Cheerful denial, with laughing or joking on totally unrelated subjects, belies the nurse's discomfort in doing that which she would rather not do.

The act may also serve to vent the hidden hostility of the nurse for the child, as a needle assumes extra force in revenge for upsetting her routine, soiling a clean bed, or being difficult for whatever reason. Being overly considerate of the pain of the child, the nurse may not be firm enough to do the task efficiently, causing the child unnecessary pain as he must be stuck again to get enough blood, or causing an IV to be restarted because restraints were not applied tightly enough.

The attitude toward inflicting pain that is most consistent with the nurse's dual roles of surrogate parent and provider of medical care is one of concerned efficiency. Those procedures causing pain are carried out as efficiently as possible, while the nurse reassures and comforts the child to lessen his perception of hurt and alienation. Speaking out for the child when others cause more pain than needed can weaken working relationships temporarily, but can also indicate the nurse's overriding concern for her patient over self and her desire that others be similarly considerate.

CHRONICALLY ILL INFANT

Not all patients in the intensive care unit are critically ill children. Many of them are in various stages of chronic illness. A few are the unfortunate infants with numerous congenital anomalies for which there is no known surgical correction.

Some infants are known as the "neonate grads"—the infants who have been in the hospital since birth, the victims of broncho-pulmonary disease or "respirator lungs." Each day the nurse must again face the challenge of weaning the infant from the ventilator and the high percentages of oxygen. It is a slow and tedious process, varying the respirator settings ever so slightly, allowing the child's pulmonary and circulatory systems to equilibrate, and then finding an unmascerated area of his heel from which to draw a blood gas determination.

Many times it is one step forward as the child tolerates the lowered oxygen level, but three steps back when mucus plugging occurs, the child's color becomes cyanotic, and the carbon dioxide level climbs as the oxygen level drops. Sometimes he is able to breathe again unassisted; sometimes the oxygen is finally lowered to room air, but the child cannot tolerate that last step. Then the painful process begins again.

Megan is one of these infants, and she has been on and off the respirator for several months. The nurses who care for her are once again striving for the better days when Megan no longer needs the respirator or the endotracheal tube. But they also know the crushing disappointment when she requires higher oxygen concentrations and longer periods for her body to adjust. At such times it's not easy to look into Megan's big, frightened eyes as she struggles for each breath.

Added to the stress of caring for these children during the time they are on the ventilator is the conflict when the unit has several of these infants, decreasing the number of beds available for emergencies and complex postoperative surgical patients. The nurse is often faced with this dilemma in working in an ICU designed to care for both the critically and the chronically ill patient.

She is torn in her priorities, knowing her attention is necessary for the critically ill child in his immediate crisis, but fearful that, if she doesn't suction the chronically ill child frequently, a mucus plug may halt the child's progress and cause him further discomfort. Yet both children are her patients and require her care and attention.

Such chronically ill children should have an intensive care area or a progressive care unit specifically devoted to them, with nurses who enjoy caring for them and who cope well with the stresses they present. Slow day-to-day progress, if any at all, the same patient for weeks or months at a time, and the all too numerous setbacks of caring for these children can be very exhausting even to the most creative nurse. The nurse working with chronic patients, in particular, deserves the opportunity for periodic relief from the demands of their care.

CHRONICALLY ILL CHILDREN IN CRISIS

When a physical crisis arises, children with chronic illnesses are often admitted to the ICU. These are the patients the nurse sees admitted time and time again, until she can't help but question: "Is it worth it?" "Will he make it through this crisis and, if he does, how long will it be until the next?" "What kind of life is this for anyone, particularly a child?"

And yet, some of these children, like Lori, age 8, with chronic leukemia, are so very eager to get their hospitalization over and to get on with the business of living. Whenever Lori comes in, everyone's spirits are lifted. Her zest for life is catching, and it renews one's hope that this admission will be another remission, and that very soon there will be a cure.

But there are also the children whose illness has left them tired and demoralized. Their bodies are emaciated and ravaged, either by the disease itself or the attempts to cure it. Their every breath is an excrutiating effort. They have a haunted look in their eyes.

Though taking care of these chronically ill patients can be very reassuring, it is not without its difficulties and tensions. The nurse must remember that this child, perhaps more than any other sick child, is a member of a family. Chronic illness takes its toll on many families and all too often causes their destruction. The nurse shares the burden of the child's illness, as well as its impact on the family.

In coping with the child and his chronic illness, the relationship of the nurse and the child's family can be a good source of mutual support, but it is not without pitfalls. If the nurse becomes too emotionally involved with the child's and the family's problems, she ceases to be the professional who must guide them and help them cope with the child's illness.

Also, the child's parents and family, who spend so much of their time at the hospital, become so versed in hospital routines and procedures that they deprive the nurse of her usual defenses. She cannot employ any of the "stalling" techniques or medical euphemisms to put them off until she herself can better cope with the situation.

Inevitably, there will be the time when the nurse must come to terms with the death of a favorite child. It may be one she has come to know and love through the years or perhaps only for a few months or weeks. The sense of loss and frustration is very real and may be intermingled with a sense of guilt. The nurse might feel that she didn't do enough, while regretting a wish that the child would die to end his painful struggle.

If there are several of these children who die in a relatively short span of time, the nurse may be hard-pressed to cope with the intensity of such feelings. The opportunity to spend time away from the ICU may be very helpful in replenishing the dwindling reserve of this nurse's resources.

THE COMATOSE CHILD

Caring for the comatose child in the ICU requires a special kind of nurse, particularly if the child arrives in a coma. She hasn't had the opportunity to see the special light in his eyes or his own unique smile. She doesn't have the advantage of knowing his personality. The nurse in this situation strives to respond to the needs of someone she doesn't know. And she may not receive any positive reinforcement for her efforts for some time, if ever.

Because the comatose patient does not respond personally to anything that the nurse does, she can adopt any attitude she chooses in their one-way interaction. She may project personality characteristics onto the child because the child reminds her of her own child, or of a brother, sister, or friend. If the nurse cannot cope with the comatose patient as a person, she may find herself becoming very cold toward him and dehumanizing the child to the level of an object. When there is still no response many weeks after admission, the nurse may tend to isolate the child and pretend he isn't there.

In working with the families of comatose children, the nurse is caught in a very awkward and stressful position. The experienced nurse knows that the longer a patient remains comatose the less chance he has of waking up, and she can readily recognize the movements and responses that are only spinal reflexes. She believes there is no hope, but is obligated to fulfill her nursing tasks as if there were. She has to maintain this attitude for the sake of the parents and family.

On the other hand, the family believes the nurse is unrealistic and heartless when she tries to be honest and straightforward with them in the face of the child's continuing lack of response. Nurses who care for these children need all the support they can get, as well as opportunity to ventilate their ambivalent feelings toward the child.

Mark was a ten-year-old boy who was involved in a car accident that claimed the lives of his parents and a younger sister. Another younger sister survived the crash with a fractured arm and some minor injuries. She was hospitalized in another state close to the home of their guardian. Mark was transferred to this ICU in a coma, with multiple trauma and fractures.

In the beginning there was physically much to do for Mark—maintain an airway, monitor vital signs, control hemorrhage, combat infection, treat for shock, maintain alignment, etc.—but Mark's care couldn't stop there. Because there was the chance for neurological improvement, Mark's nurses had to talk to him during the long weeks and months he was hospitalized. They had to rely solely on their own hope that one day he would respond.

They had to listen to Mark, too, though for many weeks there was no response. But one day when Mark's stepsister was with him, telling him that his parents and sister were killed in the car accident, Mark made his first audible response. His eyes were not the only ones in the room filled with tears.

It was a long time before Mark was able to make any further response, and his care was very exhausting. Mark was totally dependent on the nurse for all of his bodily functions. It was physically impossible for one nurse to move this once healthy boy, who was now "dead weight," in order to maintain good circulation and prevent skin breakdown.

Once Mark began to stabilize, the urinary catheter and IVs were discontinued. The nasogastric tube was no longer used for drainage of stomach contents, but as a means of providing a blenderized nourishment. With the restoration of bowel function, there was the unavoidable and distasteful task of changing diapers on a not-so-small and not-so-lightweight patient. In eight weeks the fractures had finally healed and the casts were removed. Now came the additional burden of preventing contractures and regaining full range of motion.

These and many other nursing functions were physically tiring. It was psychologically draining because, during these months, there was no response at all from Mark. With no positive reinforcement of her efforts, the nurse had to rely on inner reserves alone in order to get through the seemingly endless hours on each shift. Each of the nurses who cared for Mark had to draw many times on her best coping mechanisms in order to continue.

Today, Mark is living with close friends who have become his foster family, and has only some residual muscle weakness that eventually should be corrected. For Mark's nurses, there is the memory of a happy ending to a very difficult time, and the dread of caring for the next comatose patient, who may or may not ever respond.

DEATH AND DYING

Childhood is a time of growth, of process; a time of thinking new thoughts and doing new things; it is a time of beginnings. Everything that enters the world of the child becomes a lasting part of it, a starting point for new beginnings that lead to yet others in a seemingly endless chain of possibilities.

The death of a child is the death of possibility, an abortive end to development where there was barely a beginning. It is this loss of potential, both for the child and for those caring for him, that makes the death of children all the more tragic and difficult to deal with.

Parents are the society's agents for molding the potential of its children. By example and precept, they teach the child what is right, correct him when he is wrong, and provide the emotional and physical security in which the child can safely grow to adulthood. From parents come the care and stimulus for the child to become that which he can be: in return, they enjoy the progress of his growth and accomplishments. A child's sickness, hospitalization, and death deprive parents of their control and position as child rearers. For them, death is not only loss, but personal failure, as they are forced to surrender first their responsibilities and ultimately their child.

The basic goal of medical care is the life of its patients. Only recently and hestitatingly has medicine come to relate to death and dying in a systematic manner. The assumption has been implicit that if everything proper is done and no mistakes are made, the patient will not only live, but recover a reasonable state of health. Few nurses and doctors receive training on how to react when this does not occur. A natural response is to view death as failure on the part of those involved in the patient's care—a direct question of their competence—with all of the accompanyng feelings of anger, guilt, and sadness.

The nurse in intensive care is constantly faced with the loss of objects of affection, as patients inevitably leave, through transfer, discharge, or death. The need for emotional recovery and reinvestment is continual, but is most necessary when a patient dies and the nurse cannot help being personally involved.

Each patient represents an investment of the nurse's time, energy, and technical skills. In a profession whose hallmark is caring, the nurse is likely to make a definite emotional investment in each patient as well. Identification with a child makes the nursing care easier and more considerate, but it also makes the nurse's attachment stronger and more difficult to break when the child dies.

Death is a tacit allegation that all of the nurse's efforts were in vain. Accustomed to equating success with a patient's getting well enough to be transferred out of ICU, the nurse may take as a personal affront the patient who remains only to die. It is as if she is being spited for her work and would have been better off to do nothing at all.

Perhaps most difficult is the patient who is dying or brain dead, but who must be cared for as if there were still every chance of recovery. Todd, age 11, was on a weekend swimming outing before entering sixth grade in the fall, when an undertow carried him from knee-deep water into the middle of the river. It was twenty minutes before he was pulled from the water and resuscitated; he arrived at the hospital with pupils fixed and dilated, though his pulse was strong and regular.

For eight days he endured, with his parents interpreting as improvement his irregular, but adequate, breathing and removal from the respirator, and later his first movements since admission, which were, in fact, decerbrate posturing. While the nursing staff continued to give routine care and carried out what many considered to be hopeless heroics ordered by physicians, they also attempted to convince the family of the reality of a situation that most of them felt was doomed from the beginning.

When Todd died, his family left, drained and demoralized, and the nurses had nothing but emotional frustration to show for their work. In this type of situation it is important to avoid equating the success of nursing measures with patient health and improvement. More reasonable goals, such as giving good physical care regardless of prognosis, while focusing on support for the patient's family, can keep from making a difficult situation even more so.

The parents of the child in intensive care must make many sacrifices in their relationship with that child. They can no longer protect the child from pain and discomfort, and their position as sources of knowledge and authority has been lost to hospital personnel. Their feelings of helplessness, guilt, and grief may be displayed as hostility toward the nursing staff, but they are more likely to foster close relationships with the nurses, who provide information and reassurance, and who must be counted on to care for the child as his parents are no longer able to do.

In pediatrics, caring for the child in the context of the family is an essential part of complete care. The nurse's position as real or potential parent aids in providing the family with sympathy and support. The critically ill child who does not respond to the best medical efforts is frustrating to the nurse, who, like each member of the treatment team, gives care and attention for the satisfactions and rewards received in return. A child's death represents treatment failure, and the nurse strives to cope with feelings of impotence and guilt by reinvesting unrewarded emotional involvement with the child. The most natural object for this change of concern is the child's family.

Jennifer was a 16-year-old girl who had been followed at Children's Hospital since she was diagnosed with congenital heart disease at the age of two. Her parents were divorced many years ago, and she lived with her mother, to whom she was very close. Because of her many admissions to the hospital over the years, Jennifer and her mother became very special to the nurses in the cardiac area where she was always admitted.

Outside of a few close friends, the main support for Jennifer and her mother came from these nurses, for Jennifer's father had rejected her as being pampered and babied by the mother and Jennifer's older sister had also been alienated by the special care and attention Jennifer had needed all her life.

During the end of Jennifer's last admission for intractable congestive heart failure, a nurse was with her mother continuously because of the mother's fear of being alone when Jennifer died. As the result of seeing a television special on organ transplants, Jennifer had asked that her body be given to medical science, and it was the nurses who supported her mother in the decision to do so. It was also a nurse who was with Jennifer the evening she died and, while her mother was at supper, was able to make out Jennifer's semicomatose words, "Please let me go, I'm tired of suffering."

An hour later, when Jennifer died with her mother and a nurse in attendance, it was a great relief for both not to see her suffer anymore. Over the last week before Jennifer's death, the emotional stress for the nurses had been so great that they would suddenly burst out crying at work or at home for no apparent reason. They had carried the double burden of their own anguish and that of providing support for Jennifer's mother.

At Jennifer's death, and later at her funeral service, there were no more tears from the nurses, who were saying a final good-bye to Jennifer and telling her mother how much they cared about her and her daughter. By this time, both the mother and the nurses were well along in the grief process and were grateful for the mutual release their friendship had provided.

This type of supportive relationship between a child's nurses and his family can be of benefit to both, as both struggle to cope with a situation they cannot control. The nurse soon learns that feelings of helplessness and frustration are natural in dealing with death, but that recognizing and sharing these feelings with others can be the first step toward their resolution. Unable to enjoy the rewards of helping the child, the nurse can still preserve feelings of value and utility by helping the child's family.

The danger in developing personal, but nonprofessional, relationships with a child's family is in the binding that can occur on both sides. To the child's parents, the nurse will ever be a reminder of the death of their child, and if they cannot achieve emotional distance from the nurse as well as the child, the natural process of grieving cannot be carried to completion. For the nurse, the child's family is a reminder of treatment failure, a reminder not only of being deprived of the feelings of worth and gratification enjoyed when treatment is successful, but of the powerlessness so often felt when death is present.

Following the child's death, the nurse needs to turn her attention to the care of the other patients and families, just as the child's family needs to begin the difficult business of reestablishing day-to-day life in the absence of their loved one. There is no longer any reason, or even any possibility, of maintaining the intimate relationship created out of mutual concern for the child. Attempts at doing so are usually uncomfortable to both parties and may prevent the process of mourning from coming to an end.

If the nurse has made strong and well-received emotional attachments, attending the funeral or memorial service can be a satisfying way to express her sympathy and concern. It may also be a final act of atonement for the guilt of failing in her accepted task of sustaining life. A card of appreciation from the child's family can also be a reassuring end to the relationship, since it tells the nursing staff that their efforts were of value and appreciated even though the child died, and that the family has begun to accept the child's death.

STRESS FROM WITHIN

Amidst all the external pressures that come to bear on an ICU nurse are those that are inherent in the individual nurse.

The nurse who has children of her own and is working in a pediatric ICU may harbor several mixed emotions. Gratitude for her own healthy child; anger at the parents of a child hospitalized for abuse or ingestion; fear that her child may develop a chronic illness; anxiety that she may carry an infectious disease home; and empathy for the parents of the critically ill child are but a few of the feelings she may experience. The nurse who has no children may be too frightened of the illnesses and suffering of the children she cares for to want children of her own.

When the patient census is high and the majority of patients are critically ill, the nurse is often frustrated. The physical needs of the patients are so numerous that she must neglect their psychological and emotional needs. If, however, the nurse allows her frustration to overcome her, she may miss a brief opportunity for patting a hand or shoulder, cuddling a baby after a painful procedure, or smiling and offering words of comfort to the child or his parents as she bustles about, fulfilling her tasks. Accepting the hesitant offer of a less experienced co-worker or a parent to assist in some way can be very effectively used by the creative nurse. Many parents are eager for the chance to help with some part of their child's care, no matter how trivial it may seem.

During these times, the nurse has little chance to attend to her personal needs. The expected break period becomes a figment of her imagination. Leisurely meals are a definite luxury. In-service training or workshops to increase her knowledge or refresh her memory must be attended during precious off-duty time.

Fulfilling the teaching needs for parents, families, or the older child is haphazard or may need to be accomplished in overtime, which further infringes on the nurse's personal plans and activities.

Every nurse has her own priorities and goals in life. These may be in direct opposition to her loyalty and responsibilities to her job. She may work to provide the sole or necessary additional support for herself and her family. She may try to further her education, in order to become a better nurse and enhance her eligibility for a more challenging position and a higher rate of pay. For this nurse, there just isn't enough time, and the long hours may take their toll in sickness or exhaustion.

In trying to cope with these many pressures that are an inescapable part of her life, a nurse can very easily "burn out." The head nurse must be attuned to the signs and symptoms of her staff nurses becoming overwhelmed by one or a combination of these stresses and must be able to provide a measure of relief for their sake as well as for that of their patients.

For the head nurse, too, there are tensions that she personally brings to the position. Her conflicts come from being chosen as a head nurse because of her clinical performance as a staff nurse. She now has to abandon this and travel a somewhat different track. Many times she is caught in the middle, trying both to appease her staff and to please administration. The head nurse must redefine her own goals and realize that her expertise must be directed and developed now as a manager and not as the clinician that she used to be. She also must develop her own support systems in trying to help her staff nurses cope with their many stresses.

ADMINISTRATION

In any hospital organization when a nurse becomes frustrated, it is usually heard, "They just don't know what it's like down here for us—how hard it really is." "They" refers to the hospital administrators and, as always, the person or persons absent from the immediate situation become the scapegoat and must bear the brunt of the complaint.

There are several contradictions in the common administrative attitude. For example, the head nurse is chosen from the ranks of the staff nurses because of her clinical expertise, but is expected to abandon her clinical practice and function effectively as a manager, with little or no preparation. Staff nurses are encouraged to continue their education for degrees in nursing, but very little is done to make exceptions in scheduling to accommodate school requirements.

Administration expects nurses to give the best care possible, preferably with as few supplies as possible and the least cost to the hospital in order to function within a budget. However, little information is given to staff nurses about the budgeting process in such a large corporation.

There are as many contradictions in the staff nurses' attitudes regarding administration. They complain that administration rarely comes down to their level to see what is "really happening." When someone from the administrative level does put in an appearance on the patient floors, the staff nurses feel very uncomfortable and express their distrust by remarking, "What are they doing down here? Don't they think we're doing our jobs right?"

Some staff nurses are very disappointed when they are not fully reimbursed for their education in addition to a regular salary with fringe benefits, particularly when, for these same nurses, education takes precedence over their job responsibilities.

Because staff nurses do not have to concern themselves with paying for supplies or financing new equipment and repairing the old, some are oblivious to the high cost of medical supplies or the problem of acquiring money to purchase them.

NURSE–PHYSICIAN

One of the greatest sources of stress for the nurse in the pediatric ICU grows out of the working relationships with physicians. Since most pediatric hospitals are affiliated with teaching centers, there is usually a mixture of medical students, interns, and residents as well as staff physicians. Maintaining the proper working relationship with each of them, while providing the best care for her patients, is a continual challenge for the nurse.

Differences in judgment between physician and nurse are common, particularly with new house officers or those on the pediatric rotation of an adult service. Some of the physicians are sure to be inexperienced, unfamiliar with pediatrics, or both, and it often falls to the nurse to decide which orders are appropriate and when outside help is needed. Drug dosages, for example, are a frequent source of error and must be calculated from the child's weight in kilograms. The nurse giving an adult-maintenance Digoxin dose of 0.25 mg. to a 20-kg. child would be just as much at fault as the doctor who ordered it rather than a typical 0.08 mg.

Although the nurse may be more experienced and knowledgeable than the physician she is working with, she is violating the traditional passive nursing role by telling the doctor what to do or giving advice on patient management. Paradoxically, she must be the final patient advocate, and making certain her patients receive what she believes to be right is very much a nursing responsibility. If she cannot tactfully convince the physician that his decision needs to be changed, she may need to go to his resident or even the attending physician for resolution.

Having a physician available on short notice is a requirement of all ICUs. For medical patients at Children's Hospital, this is seldom a problem since pediatricians are always nearby. Specialty services that have offices elsewhere, such as surgery, chest surgery, ENT, orthopedics, and plastic surgery, must depend upon the nurse to observe their patients and report any problems. This sharpens the nurse's diagnostic skills, but may also leave her without guidance in an emergency situation.

The day following her tetralogy of Fallot repair, two-year-old Theresa began having arrhythmias. With the chest surgeons all in the O.R., the nurse reached the chest intern on-call, who was in his first rotation and had little experience in pediatric heart problems. Theresa's pediatric intern was available, but the chest surgeons had previously made it clear that no orders were to be written on their patients without specific approval. After considerable delay and much anxiety on the part of the nurse and Theresa's mother, the pediatric resident was persuaded to intervene and begin treatment. The chest surgeons were upset, but reluctantly agreed that the right things had been done.

There may be several services involved in some complicated patients, each writing orders and each with different thoughts about managing the patient's care. This can prove very frustrating for the nurse when the physicians contradict and cancel each other's orders. She is obliged to act as the messenger between services, as complaints and other comments are often directed to her rather than to the physicians involved. When parents wish to speak to a physician about their child, the nurse must decide who is the most appropriate one to do so.

The nurse is bound to the ICU for most of her shift, while the physician may come or go as desired. Being uncomfortable with a patient's impending death, insecurity about treatment, or difficulty in dealing with a child's family may all be reasons for the physician to avoid being in the ICU. The nurse is faced with doing what she can by herself or attempting to persuade the physician to become more actively involved.

NURSE—NURSE

The many stresses and responsibilities in an ICU tend to foster a strong group feeling among its nurses. Physically, the intensive care units are set apart from the rest of the hospital. They receive the most acutely ill children and the most involved surgeries. ICU nurses must handle complicated equipment and perform technical procedures in a variety of acute situations. They must deal effectively with the very sick child and his family. And they must be able to work closely with other nurses and professionals at times when feelings and personalities are most likely to clash. Nurses able to meet these demands consider themselves part of a special group and take pride in having a difficult job and doing it well.

The nurse's feelings of professional identity and worth are directly tied to the group identity, particularly if she is a new graduate or new to intensive care. From fellow staff nurses, she learns the needed technical skills, as well as the group norms of how to interact with everyone from the housekeeping person to the hospital director. Typically understaffed, the ICU welcomes new nurses and usually responds with support and encouragement as they learn their new role. If a new nurse does not meet the group's expectations, however, it can mean censure and a difficult work situation.

Patient care, as well as equipment, supplies, and space, are all shared among nurses. Although each nurse has her own patients, she is dependent upon other nurses for coverage during meals and emergencies and for assistance in tasks she cannot accomplish alone. It is essential that she work well with others on the staff, both for the sake of her patients and for her own sense of job satisfaction. Group acceptance demands cooperation.

The group is also the source of many social relationships, as the most understanding friend an ICU nurse can have is usually another ICU nurse. Extracurricular social activities, such as parties, baby showers, or having a drink after work, all serve to reinforce the group and provide outlets for sharing work experiences and difficulties. Incidents involving doctors, support personnel, or even fellow nurses are related, with emphasis on group perceptions of the absent person's mistakes. There is much more opportunity for criticism than for praise of good work, and judgment of others further serves to define the group and its expectations.

Nurses on regular patient divisions may be viewed by the ICU staff as having lower status and less competence. Bobby, an infant with a new tracheostomy, did well enough to be transferred from ICU, only to return a week later with worsening pneumonia. His readmission brought comments about floor nurses "not knowing how to suction," and "We shouldn't have gotten this kid back."

Nurses outside the ICU may indeed look upon its staff as elite and particularly competent. The ICU is the most attractive unit in the hospital; it has the most "status," the most deaths, the most burned or abused or nearly drowned children, whose stories appeared on the evening news. Other nurses must come to the ICU nurse to satisfy their curiosity about such events or to get information on their own patients who have come to the ICU. The ICU nurse may be used as a reference for the more technical aspects of patient care that are not practiced regularly by floor nurses. But they also point out that the ICUs get the best equipment, the closest attention from doctors, and the most staff, which is especially evident when there are few patients requiring intensive care.

The very environment of an "intensive" care unit tends to promote tension and disagreement. Yet the work itself leaves no time for their resolution, and informal group norms further discouarge the expression of conflict. Interpersonal anger may instead be expressed towards patients or their families. It may find release in after-work activities with other ICU nurses, whom the nurse feels are the only ones who can really appreciate what has happened. Perhaps more often, stresses find expression in the nurse's personal life. Family members or close friends may be asked to share the distressing story of the child who died that day, or may be the recipients of the displaced anger for a doctor or co-worker, which could not be vented on the job.

Expectations of group loyalty may present other conflicts with the nurse's private hours. Refusal to attend group social activities can be seen as criticism, while the nurse may simply wish to fulfill responsibilities to family and friends. When the nurse is ill, she may feel obligated to come to work anyway, rather than let others down and increase their workload. Conversely, similar guilt feelings can arise when the nurse is asked to work extra hours when doing so would destroy personal plans.

STRESS REDUCTION

A number of papers have been written describing the unique stresses experienced by the nurses working in intensive care units.[1–7] Most of these papers make suggestions for alleviating such stresses. The possible approaches may be listed under three headings: (1) those affecting the management of the ICU environment; (2) those dealing with the individual nurse; and (3) those involving ICU nurses as a group.

Making the best use of available resources in the ICU is a difficult task. Management must be objective and controlled, rather than crisis-oriented, as patient care must be at times. In an effort to keep decision-making as close as possible to actual nursing, at Children's Hospital the patient care managers (formerly called head nurses) are given much autonomy. Shortly after being appointed, the new manager is sent through a program that teaches basic management principles. Later other opportunities are made available to develop such skills. Each manager is responsible for her area's budget, interviewing and hiring new staff nurses, staff performance evaluations, and all decisions related to managing patient care on her unit, subject to final approval by the director of patient care.

Careful attention to the use of support personnel, to supplies, physical environment, and staff scheduling can greatly reduce potential stresses for the ICU nurse, particularly if she is encouraged to work with the manager toward their recognition and resolution. The involvement of staff in decision-making and change[8] can contribute to greater job interest and satisfaction, improved communication, and better patient care.[9]

It is not always possible to change or eliminate the causes of stress in the ICU, so mediating its effects is a necessity. Each individual has his or her own techniques for the management of stress. When the nurse's usual coping mechanisms do not provide a consistent, reality-oriented, reduction of stress, other methods must be actively pursued. The nurse who is overly upset each time a child dies might get help by exploring her feelings about death with a counselor or religious worker. Long-term, constructive methods for coping with stress can include talking with supportive others, prayer or meditation, drawing on past experiences, physical exercise, and deciding on alternate ways to handle the stressful situation.[10]

The method that most directly addresses the stresses of ICU nursing as they occur is the holding of regular group meetings with a knowledgeable facilitator.[3,11] All staff members are encouraged to attend, and discussion is limited to personal and interpersonal concerns that are directly related to patient care. The same forces that define the group so sharply can contribute to its effectiveness in problem solving when constructively channeled.

Cassem and Hackett[6] have summarized the steps necessary for successful group resolution of stress: "(1) identification and acknowledgment of feelings; (2) sharing of these feelings; (3) review of the experience with criticism, support, and praise; (4) followed by integration of what is learned with application in future experience." In those settings where such a group process was employed, strong support has been given to its value for both nursing staff[6,11] and patients.[12]

To help the new nurse become familiar with the emotional, as well as the technical, aspects of the ICU, her orientation could include exploration with the group leader of typically stressful situations: the child who is brain-dead; hostile parents; the inexperienced doctor; requests to work extra shifts; the need to hurt patients; cardiac arrests; making mistakes. Through role playing and discussion, she might gain an understanding of the feelings involved and possible ways to cope with them.

SUMMARY

The staff of a pediatric intensive care unit is faced with considerable stress in fulfilling their duties. A complex and often ceaseless work load, the need to inflict pain on children who may be unable to respond, and the repeated treatment failure of death all strain the nurse's ability to remain and to provide consistent care. Clear communication with doctors, families, and other nurses is inhibited by individual stresses and the amount and urgency of patient needs. This further increases the nurse's own need for support and resolution of conflict. Yet her responsibilities and informal group norms discourage withdrawal or the open expression of disagreements. The nurse may be forced to adopt inadequate coping mechanisms, such as displacement or denial, in order to deal with feelings that the ICU does not allow her to express in other ways.

Means for achieving on-going stress reduction for the ICU nurse can include her participation in its management, active concern for her own well-being, and regular group meetings with a skilled facilitator who would also conduct psychological orientation for new employees.

Nurses working in intensive care units, whether pediatric or adult, have to be particularly competent in recognizing and dealing with the problems of patients and families[13,14] who are under a great deal of stress. The challenge of providing physical and emotional support under trying conditions is a crucial part of the satisfactions as well as the frustrations of ICU nursing. With proper guidance, the same energy and understanding that allow ICU nurses to give superior patient care can be used effectively to reduce their own stresses.[5] The result can be an atmosphere that is not only less stressful, but more conducive to meeting the needs of nurse and patient alike.

REFERENCES

1. Hay D, Oken D: The Psychological Stresses of Intensive Care Unit Nursing. Psychosom Med 34: 109–117, 1972

2. Jacobson SP: Stressful Situations for Neonatal Intensive Care Nurses. MCN 3: 144–150, 1978

3. Vreeland V, Ellis GL: Stresses on the Nurse in an Intensive Care Unit. JAMA 208: 332–334, 1969

4. Michaels DR: Too Much in Need of Support to Give Any? Am J Nurs 71: 1932–1935, 1971

5. Bilodeau CB: The Nurse and Her Reactions to Critical-Care Nursing. Heart and Lung 2: 358–362, 1973

6. Cassem NH, Hackett TP: Stress on the Nurse and Therapist in the Intensive-Care Unit and the Coronary Care Unit. Heart and Lung 4: 252–259, 1975

7. Melia KM: The Intensive Care Unit—A Stress Situation? Nurs Times 73(5): 17–20 (center) 1977

8. Kinney M, Millington P, Jackson BS: Planned Change in the Critical Care Unit. Heart and Lung 7: 85–90, 1978

9. Niessner P: Participative Management in the ICU. Supervisor Nurse 9(3): 41–44, 1978

10. Bell JM: Stressful Life Events and Coping Methods in Mental-Illness and Wellness Behaviors. Nurs Res 26: 136–141, 1977

11. Simon NM, Whiteley S: Psychiatric Consultation with MICU Nurses: The Consultation Conference as a Working Group. Heart and Lung 6: 497–521, 1977

12. Dubovsky SL, Getto CJ, Gross SA, et al: Impact on Nursing Care and Mortality: Psychiatrists on the Coronary Care Unit. Psychos Med 18(3): 18–28, 1977

13. Epperson MM: Families in Sudden Crisis: Process and Intervention in a Critical Care Center. Soc Work Health Care 2: 265–273, 1977

14. Gardner D, Stewart N: Staff Involvement with Families of Patients in Critical Care Units. Heart and Lung 7: 105–110, 1978

CHAPTER **9**

Psychological Aspects of MICU-CCU Nursing: Patient Problems

Nathan M. Simon

The MICU is a direct outgrowth of the original ICU concept in that it has become the treatment site for a heterogeneous group of seriously ill (medical) patients. In medical centers with separate Coronary Care Units (CCU) and Respiratory Intensive Care Units (RICU), the MICU patients are the critically ill with multiple systems diseases (combined cardiac, pulmonary, neurologic, and renal problems), more virulant forms of collagen disease, life-threatening infections, blood dyscrasias, acute renal failure, certain malignancies, and transfers from other units such as Surgical Intensive Care Units (SICU). In smaller hospitals or those without a separate CCU, there will be a significant number of acute myocardial infarctions (MIs) or possible MIs admitted. The CCU admits primarily patients with acute MIs or possibility of MI and other serious cardiac illnesses.

Patient diagnoses influence the mood of the unit. The MI patient usually has a short stay (4 to 5 days), a relatively good outcome for the immediate future, and is conscious and communicative. The non-MI patient usually has a longer stay, relatively poor outcome for both the immediate and distant future, and impaired consciousness and communication. The nurse is in a paradoxical situation. The patient from whom she can receive the most direct gratification, both in immediate feedback and in the pleasure of seeing her nursing skills lead to an improvement, is also the one with whom she will have the briefest contact and the more superficial relation. Conversely, the nurse will usually form more intense relationships with the sicker, longer-staying patient and the patient's family, but also will find much less direct gratification from the patient because of the patient's passivity relative to the nurse's great activity, the patient's impaired ability to communicate, and the nurse's need to acknowledge that, for all of her professional skills, the patient will most likely die.

There is intrinsically more strain on the nursing staff of the MICU than on the staff of the CCU. They are faced with hopeless situations that stretch over long periods of time. Death rates are higher; the repetitive experience of loss and failure is more frequent. The optimistic tone that is characteristic of the CCU is diluted considerably in the MICU.

The discussion that follows will consider patients and nurses in both MICU and CCU because, though the environments are in some respects dissimiliar, most of the psychological issues are the same, even though the differences in clinical problems lead to varying emphasis on specific issues.

ANXIETY

Anxiety typically is most intense and most frequently observed in the earliest days of hospitalization for patients on the MICU or CCU. Even patients who claim that they are not fearful may be anxious, as attested to by high catecholomine output in patients identified as deniers.[1] The most obvious cause of anxiety in acute life-threatening illness is the fear of death. Patients who initially admit to, and openly express, anxiety experience a decrease in anxiety over time. They also are more likely to accurately identify improvement in their health status relative to the day of admission.[2]

Valium and other chemical agents of the same group are effective in helping to manage the acute phases of anxiety. Chemical agents alone are less helpful in chronic anxiety states. Also these antianxiety drugs frequently cannot be used in patients where concern about central nervous system depression is important. Patients with pulmonary disease and on respirators make up a large part of this group of patients.

Even where antianxiety drugs can be used, the nurse is still the major antianxiety agent on MICUs or CCUs. Careful support from the nursing staff is needed, in combination at times with brief psychotherapy and/or specific behavioral programs where appropriate behavior is shaped by using an operant to reward the patient (uninterrupted stay in the room with the patient, a backrub, extended visiting by family, etc).

Example: A 61-year-old married woman, who had a myocardial infarction, underwent a tracheotomy because of a respiratory crisis shortly after admission and was on a ventilator. The patient was extremely demanding and anxious. She called the nurses constantly. Her husband's and brother's visits made the patient more anxious. They openly expressed worry and concern about the patient while they were in the room and wondered aloud why she was not doing better and why the nurses and doctors were not doing anything for her. The nurses limited family visiting, which produced a decrease in anxiety. The patient became dependent on the ventilator and anxious about any changes made in the intermittent manditory ventilation (IMV) prescription. When she was told she was going to be weaned from the respirator, she responded with much anxiety and an angry outburst directed at the nurse who told her. The nurse accepted this in a non-critical way and was supportive, but firm. She remained with the patient for the early parts of the weaning program which, after a rather rocky first day, proceeded smoothly over the next several days until the patient was breathing without assistance.

DEPRESSION

Many writers have commented on the regularity with which depression appears on MICU and CCU patients.[3–7] In patients with MIs, the sequence is often anxiety the first day of the hospitalization followed by depression in the later days. In longer stay patients, depression is almost always a finding. The enforced passivity, the loss of self-esteem, the concern about facing the future with marked impairment, or not having any future at all, contribute to the genesis of depression. In addition, many of the patients have illnesses that produce symptoms of exhaustion, decreased energy, decreased interest, and decreased mental activities because of the physiological changes that take place (fever, electrolyte imbalance, poor brain and tissue oxygenation).

Example: A 74-year-old white single woman was admitted with severe substernal pain. There were no ECG changes and no enzyme evidence of MI. The patient was transferred off the unit, but chest pain persisted and she was transferred back to the CCU. She became increasingly depressed. Arteriograms revealed three-vessel disease with "high lesions," which she was told gave her an excellent prognosis for the bypass surgery that was recommended and to which she agreed. The patient's depression deepened after the decision for surgery was made. She expressed suicidal thoughts. She was anxious and would literally cling to the nurses who cared for her, kissing their hands frequently. She appeared confused at times, although she remained oriented. She and her family became more ambivalent about the surgery as the day approached. She had many runs of ventricular tachycardia two days prior to the surgery. However, the day before surgery she quite suddenly appeared less depressed and more optimistic. At surgery, there were no technical difficulties, but during the procedure the patient arrested and died.

This patient is an example of a group of patients who demonstrate high levels of anxiety and significant signs and symptoms of depression. These patients have a poor prognosis. Though the patient gave ample evidence of her state of distress, with open expressions of anxiety, suicidal thoughts, and runs of PVCs, more attention was paid to the locus of the vessel obstruction than to the patient's overall condition. This is a situation in which input from the nurses was not given adequate consideration by the medical staff. It is also possible that the nurses themselves did not recognize the importance of the observations they were making in their care of the patient. Ideally, a conference involving all of the professional staff could have evaluated the patient's clinical state in those days prior to surgery. Nursing staff could have taken the lead for such a conference. Careful review of the patient's responses to her illness and to the impending surgery would probably have led to a decision to postpone surgery, at least until her anxiety and depression were better controlled, or perhaps not to operate at all.

This type of situation requires a shifting of nursing care plans and types of interventions by the nursing staff. Initially, the goals would have been to help the patient to deal with the depression related to her illness and her concerns about the recommendation for surgery. At that point, reassurance, explanation of the procedures and what the future held, support by frequent contacts with the patient, and spending adequate time with the patient in discussions about the options all would have been useful. But as evidence for serious depression accumulated, the nursing approach could have been modified to include: (1) a request for a staff conference; (2) psychiatric consultation; (3) more exploration and interest in the patient's reservations about surgery; (4) a more empathic response to the extent of her fears of death; and (5) support of the patient and family in talking more openly to the physicians about the possibility of delaying the procedure until the patient's and the family's ambivalence about it were better resolved.

Depressive symptoms are a "normal" response to the MICU. Acknowledging this to the patient, with understanding, acceptance, and willingness to talk about the depressed feelings, goes far toward helping the patient live through this phase. Early patient activity, where possible, and early introduction to rehabilitative and education programs about the illness are other positive ways to help deal with the depression of the ICU. There is also some evidence that psychotherapy with MI patients started as soon as the patient is stabilized physically can cut down on the in-hospital depression and posthospital disability.[8]

Antidepressant drugs cannot be used very often on MICUs or on CCUs, although they may play a part in after-discharge treatment plans.

DELIRIUM, HALLUCINATIONS, AND DELUSIONS

Parker and Hodges[9] identified 12 episodes of delirium in 11 patients out of approximately 500 patients admitted to a 12-bed, open-ward CCU. The mean duration of symptoms was 4.5 days, but less severe episodes were of shorter duration. One case, judged mild, showed brief periods of disorientation and inappropriate behavior. The one case judged moderate demonstrated prolonged confusion, apprehension, and restlessness. Six cases, graded moderately severe, exhibited illusions, hallucinations, and paranoid ideation. Four episodes, judged severe, demonstrated combativeness and panic. There was no relationship between the extent of myocardial damage, as estimated by enzyme elevation, hypertension, cardiac failure, or other complications, and the severity of the delirium. Mean time between admission and onset of delirium was two to three days (15–96 hours range). Disorientation, usually at night, and inappropriate remarks were often the first indications. The authors urge that restraints be avoided where possible. They found phenothiazines helpful, but the best response occurred in patients who were moved to a side room or a general medical floor, where family members were allowed to stay with them for long periods of time.

The high levels of anxiety, compromised cerebral functioning due to physiological changes, and an elderly patient population combine to make hallucinations regular MICU and CCU phenomena. It is useful to attempt to understand these symptoms as a way of communicating and not just to write them off as the result of "bad blood gases."

Example: A 74-year-old man with near-end-stage chronic obstructive pulmonary disease (COPD) had been a patient in an MICU for 12 weeks. The patient had a tracheotomy and had been on a ventilator for much of this time. There was a fairly good correlation between mild confusional states and low PO_2 and high PCO_2 levels. The patient was weaned from the ventilator with difficulty. He was still on nasal oxygen. Blood gases were borderline at best. The patient, who had a very good relationship with the nurses and was liked by all of them, was told he would soon be transferred off the unit and would be able to return home. That night the patient, when his blood gases were usually worse, for the first time in the 12 weeks of hospitalization began to hallucinate. He heard FBI agents talking to him over his television set. They were trying to send messages about him to people. The FBI agents were out to get him. The hallucinations and mild disorientation occurred sporadically for a few days and then disappeared. During this time, the nurses talked with the patient about his anxiety related to discharge and he gradually seemed calmer and better organized. He was eventually discharged.

The nurse's response to this patient illustrates the accurate analysis of a problem and the instituting of an appropriate and effective nursing plan to deal with it. The unit nurses had an excellent working relationship established with this patient and his family prior to the episode described. The change in the patient's mental status was promptly noted and given serious consideration. The patient was discussed at a conference with the unit consultant psychiatrist where the importance of the patient's feelings about discharge was understood as an important stress. The nurses decided which of the nurses had the best working relationship with the patient and they were assigned to care for him in this period. They systematically took advantage of opportunities to discuss discharge, explored his anxieties about discharge, and talked in positive ways about plans for the patient's continued care after discharge.

Not all hallucinations are products of the MICU. Some are brought in by the patients.

Example: A 66-year-old widow was admitted with severe congestive heart failure. She had a history of myocardial infarction. According to the patient's older daughter, the patient had been diagnosed as a paranoid schizophrenic many years previously. This daughter described that patient as having been very "crazy" for the month prior to admission. In addition to diuretics and digitalis, the patient received 5 mgm of Valium, an 8 mgm dose of morphine sulfate, followed in three hours by a 4 mgm dose of morphine sulphate. She had a copious diuresis and slept for several hours. On awakening, she was agitated. Communicating by written notes, she repeated over and over, "They're doing it, they're doing it to me. They're trying to kill me." She vigorously resisted suctioning and had to be restrained. Her heart rate increased from 90 per minute on admission to 200 per minute. It was observed that her younger daughter's presence seemed to calm the patient considerably. The daughter remained with her for several hours until the situation stabilized. Tranquilizers were started and the endotracheal tube was removed the next day. The patient remained paranoid and delusional during her stay on the MICU.

This is another example of prompt and effective development of a nursing care plan. The initial critical work was accomplished by nursing contact with the patient's daughter at the time of admission to the ICU. History was obtained by the nurse at that time about the patient's chronic psychiatric illness. The second step was the nurse's observation of the difference in the patient's response to her two daughters and her prompt utilization of this observation to help manage the patient's anxiety.

Another frequent cause of hallucinations is medication used to treat arrythmias. Lidocaine is a primary offender. Hallucinations are often visual and can be frightening. Propranalol is also capable of producing visual hallucinations. Digitalis intoxication has visual symptoms ("yellow vision" and blurring of vision) that sometimes can be mistaken for hallucinations.

Example: A 74-year-old male was admitted to the MICU after spending two days on a regular medical nursing division. His admission diagnoses were MI and mild chronic brain syndrome. He was receiving Lidocaine by IV drip. Within hours of transfer to the MICU, he reported seeing people walking on the walls. The bed side stand also seemed to be on the wall. He told the nurse that he must be having hallucinations and that something was wrong with him. He became convinced that this was true when he noted that the orange juice was not spilling out of the glass, even though it was on top of the bed side table, which appeared to be on the wall. He realized that this did not make sense and that he was perceiving things incorrectly. After discussing this with the nurse, who was reassuring and commended him for telling her about what he saw, his anxiety decreased. With the discontinuation of the Lidocaine, the symptoms disappeared completely.

Where hallucinations, delusions, and agitation become major interferences with the overall treatment plan, it is necessary to adopt a vigorous and straightforward approach in trying to control the anxiety. Intravenous Haloperidol is an effective anti-psychotic agent that is quick-acting and can be extremely useful in helping to control severely agitated and delusional patients. Haloperidol has the advantage of being relatively fast-acting and also of producing relatively little in the way of central nervous system depression at the dosage levels used for crisis situations.[10,11] Experience with it to date indicates that it can be safely used even in patients with arrhythmias.

With all organic brain syndromes, the nurse needs to help the patient, in every way possible, to stay oriented. The strange physical environment, the multitude of new faces, the physiological effects of the illness and medications all combine to confuse and disorient the patient who has organic brain syndrome. Clear introductions, announcing one's name, repetitions of time, day, date, and place, reducing the nursing staff who have contact with the patient to the bare minimum, providing maximum contact with someone familiar and friendly (wife, husband, child) are all ways to assist the patient in remaining oriented.

ANGER

Angry outbursts or continuous anger is frequently part of some patients' adaptive response to the MICU or CCU. Hackett[12] points out that anger and complaints about nursing care are more characteristic of patients with terminal malignancies and rare in patients on CCUs. However, the angry complaints do occur on CCUs and often anger is used as a way of warding off anxiety.

Example: A 63-year-old man with severe chest pain was admitted to a MICU. His chest pain occurred immediately after a violent argument with his new supervisor at work. That patient had tried to "fire" the new supervisor because he had found that he was proceeding "illegally." The patient claimed that the supervisor physically threatened him during the argument. The ECG showed ST segment depression. Enzymes were negative for myocardial infarction. On the first hospital day, the patient was apathetic and hardly spoke. On the second day, there were a number of arrests on the unit and two deaths. Although the patient was in a single room, he was aware of the commotion on the unit and also quite aware that the nurses were not as available to him as they were on his first hospital day. He became angrily demanding. In an angry and imperious voice he accused the nurses of "bad nursing," demanded to see the head of the unit, and said he would write to the Director of the Hospital protesting his treatment.

Many times, responses of patients are difficult to predict. The patient's first day apathy was seen as a rather "usual" reaction to admission to the MICU with the possibility of having just suffered a heart attack. In retrospect, it is easy to say that the initial nursing care plan could have included more time spent with the patient and more interest and appreciation of the stress he was experiencing then. The numerous crises on the unit on the second day of the patient's stay made it impossible to institute a plan that might have avoided the angry outbursts. With more nursing time available, the plan could have included more frequent visits to the patient's room by the nurse. When the patient demonstrated interest and anxiety about the unit crisis, the nurse could have been in a position to talk with him about his concerns simply and honestly in a reassuring way. This very well may have included some open discussion of the patient's feelings about his heart attack. The nurse could, if the patient's anxiety and anger abated enough to allow him to listen to her, in a calm and reassuring way talk about the encouraging ECG and laboratory findings that were part of the patient's workup. Because ideal conditions were not present, the next consideration must be ways of responding to the patient's angry outbursts.

The first step here is to recognize anger as a coping response to: (1) the patient's "near" heart attack; (2) the anxiety aroused in the patient by the unit crisis; and (3) the anxiety aroused by his being deprived of support by the nurses. Appropriate nursing reaction could: (1) avoid angry, defensive, accusatory responses to the patient's anger; (2) acknowledge that nurses had indeed been less available to the patient during his second day of hospital stay; (3) acknowledge that the patient's upset may be due in part to his awareness of the unit crises and the anxiety that it may have caused him; and (4) make sure that nursing visits with the patient were not rushed or avoided because of the patient's anger and accusatory behavior.

Example: A 50-year-old married man with two young children was admitted to the MICU for the first time with a myocardial infarction. He had many arrythmias and was cardioverted several times in the first week of hospitalization. He was alert during several episodes of ventricular tachycardia and during the cardioversions. He was never thought to be a problem patient during that stay. Eight weeks later he was readmitted with severe chest pain. ECG and enzymes were negative. From the time he entered the unit, he distinguished himself by being as angrily obnoxious as possible. By the end of the first day, all the nurses who had contact with him labeled him a "creep." He griped angrily about everything and, even when the nurses made efforts to correct situations he complained about (room temperature, food, electrode placement), he continued to complain. On the morning of the second hospital day, he asked his doctor for permission to get up to go to the bathroom and to be disconnected from the monitor. His doctor refused. When the nurse brought his breakfast tray shortly afterward, he threw it across the room and cursed the nurse. He shouted as he told the House Officer, who came to investigate, that the tray was late, the nursing care was bad, and that he didn't like this place. The House Officer heard him out, acknowledged his upset, and made it clear that the patient's behavior was not acceptable. The patient subsided somewhat. In contacts with the same nurse, he retained an aggressive manner for the rest of the day. In response to a simple question, he would say "Yes, damn it." And when asked about chest pain, "I wouldn't tell you if I had it!" The nurse who wanted to "clobber" the patient for his behavior remained with him and did not distance herself from him. He became somewhat less aggressive as the day went on and he began to tell her about all the pressures on his job. He owned a contracting company. He talked about all the complaints he had to deal with from customers and employees about "little things," especially complaining about employees who depended upon him. The nurse was finally able to ask him if he felt frightened about being readmitted so soon after his heart attack. The patient responded, with much less anger, that he had been very scared during his first admission but that he was not scared anymore. He talked about the anxiety he experienced while he was alert during the cardioversions. While he was still abrasive and quarrelsome with the nurse and with his wife as well (who said that this was not such unusual behavior for him, although it was exaggerated), he did not have any more angry outbursts. He did insist on being discharged in three days to "take care of his business."

The nurse caring for this patient responded with great sensitivity and tact to the patient's behavior. She identified her own feeling state quickly and was able to keep it from intruding. She maintained good contact with the patient and did not avoid him because of his anger. She correctly understood that his anger was an attempt to deal with his anxiety and was in part engendered by the passivity involved in being a patient. The nurse was able to accept a more controlled form of the patient's anger as the patient's way of attempting to maintain some type of active mastery and masculine role.

SEXUAL BEHAVIOR

There is much overt sexual behavior on MICUs and CCUs that never receives official recognition. The MICU and CCU literature does emphasize that an event like an MI may be immediately interpreted by a patient as being the end of all sexual activity. However, only one brief mention of current sexual behavior by patients in the CCU and MICU was discovered in a literature search.[13] Only the dialysis unit literature recognizes its presence.[14] It is elsewhere relegated to unofficial discussions among staff members. In a routine meeting with eight MICU nurses, all of them, when asked directly, reported observing at least one episode of overt sexual behavior by a patient in the preceding three-month period. All involved male patients with female nurses.

Many of the sexual behaviors that do occur are: (1) ways of expressing, via some overt sexual act, other feelings such as anger; (2) efforts to deal with high levels of anxiety; (3) efforts to ward off feelings of helplessness; or (4) efforts to reassure himself that sexual function is not lost forever. The overt sexual behaviors seen in the MICU include masturbation, exhibitionism, attempts to fondle or paw nurses, and verbal behavior—i.e., sexual references and sexual invitations.

The masturbatory activity that is seen may not actually be masturbation to orgasm. Masturbation appears most often to be used as a way of calming and reducing tension in situations where great anxiety is present. Occasionally, it will be performed by the patient for reassurance that erections and sexual feelings are still possible. Sometimes exhibitionism is a part of a mild or moderately severe chronic brain syndrome. The patient is not as aware of self and regresses to infantile levels of gratification.

Example: A 75-year-old man had been admitted three days previously with a mild MI and congestive failure. The nurse, who was an attractive young woman, helped the patient to a chair and brought him his dinner. After dinner the patient called to have the tray cleared and to be helped back to bed. As the nurse stood in front of him giving support under his elbows, he half rose from the chain and bit her on the right breast. He smiled and gave a half laugh. Before she could even think about it the nurse hit him on the shoulder with her fist. She felt violated and humilitated. She immediately went to the charge nurse and reported what had happened. The charge nurse told the intern, who admonished the patient and told him that nurses were not to be treated that way. The patient denied he had done anything to the nurse and claimed she was lying. He said the nurse was young enough to be his daughter and did not appeal to him anyway. The nurse refused to go back into the patient's room for the rest of his stay on the unit.

The above example is a situation in which it is easy to understand the nurse's spontaneous reaction. However, it is also important to understand what was going on with the patient. This situation is one in which the nurse needs to clearly establish with the patient what is acceptable behavior. Also, ideally, it should be done in a way without disrupting the overall nursing relationship with the patient.

Sometimes sexual behavior is quite clearly part of a long-standing aggressive and hostile way of interacting with women.

Example: A 56-year-old man, recovering from an MI, constantly made salacious remarks when the nurses came into the room while his wife was there. He would proposition the nurses and suggest that they jump into bed with him and he would compare his wife to them unfavorably. The entire experience was embarrassing to his wife, which was the primary intent. The patient had a long-standing, passive-aggressive relationship with his wife, which he continued at the hospital. Without hostility, the nurse who was involved in this initial display talked to the patient in the presence of the patient's wife about the hostile and depreciating aspects of the patient's remarks. She identified it, quite correctly, as not at all flattering to her, but as an embarrassment and attack on his wife. After the nurse dealt with the situation, the patient's behavior changed and he did not repeat it again during his stay on the CCU.

Sometimes sexuality can be used in a way to obtain some control over a situation.

Example: A 23-year-old male quadraplegic, who was admitted with huge infected decubiti, bladder and kidney infections, and bacterial pneumonia, used a never-ending stream of obscene sexual language with women nurses. He was also grandiose. He would tell stories about wild sexual parties he had participated in before the injury that had resulted in his spinal cord transection. He was attempting, by his language, which was the only motor area left in his complete control, to establish some dominance and control over the nurses on whom he was totally dependent. He was trying to frighten them, to intimidate them, and to awe them all at the same time.

The nursing plan for this patient evolved out of understanding that, for this patient, greatly limited physically, emotionally, and socially, and with very few adaptive resources available to him even before his injury, the sex talk and obscenity had become a major coping device. The nurses' anger at him decreased somewhat with this issue clarified, although they found it best to rotate on a daily basis the nurses assigned to his care. Using male nursing staff also provoked less in the way of obscenities from the patient and less provocative talk. The nurses made it clear that they wanted to make contact with him in ways other than as objects of his verbal abuse, and they made attempts to empathize with his anger.

TRANSFER FROM THE UNIT

In two of the examples previously used, an important element was the patient's response to actual or possible transfer from the MICU. Transfer is not an innocuous event to the patient. Hackett[3] found that over 25% of the patients had a negative response to transfer. While many patients see transfer as a sign of improvement and greater freedom, about one in four will experience transfer as a threat. The loss of security that comes from the intensive nursing care, the monitors, and the frequent visits from physicians are important matters to patients who have experienced life-threatening illness.

Klein[15] studied a series of 14 patients with MI, transferred from a CCU to a general medical ward, by clinical observations and urinary catecholamine excretion. The first seven patients were transferred without any special preparation or post-transfer planning. In this group, five out of the seven showed increases in catecholamines after transfer. All of these five developed major complications (re-infarction, pericarditis, ventricular tachycardia, coronary insufficiency), and one died with ventricular fibrillation. The second group of seven patients was prepared from admission for the possibility of transfer. A nurse from the CCU followed them to the general medical ward and spent one hour a day with them there, and one physician was assigned to them for the entire hospital stay. Two of these patients had a rise in urinary catechalomines and five did not. Only one patient developed a complication after transfer (organic brain syndrome). Klein's study makes an extremely strong case for careful preparation for transfer off the unit and suggests that Hackett underestimated the scope and severity of the problem.

Example: A 63-year-old man was admitted to a CU with an MI. After one and one half days on the unit, the infarction extended. The patient had two days of cardiac rhythm instability and then did well physiologically. However, the patient became very dependent on the nurses. He became afraid of any physical activity. The nurses worked actively with the patient and the family who visited regularly. They began the cardiac rehabilitation program and were supportive of the patient as he began to become active again. The patient was told he was going to be transferred. As the day of transfer approached, the patient talked to the nurses about "seeing angels" and he asked if the nurses "knew anyone in heaven." The nurses responded with reassurance, talked with him about his anxiety about leaving the unit, and told him they understood that he was telling them he felt it was premature.

This example also illustrates that not everything that sounds like a hallucination is one. The patient was talking in metaphors to the nurses, letting them know he was afraid of dying, and trying to make it clear to them that, if he was transferred from the unit, he would die. His way of talking to them about "seeing angels and knowing people in heaven" was his attempt to enlist their help in his cause, receive their sympathy, and arouse their guilt.

CARDIAC ARRESTS—PATIENT DEATHS

Even the patient in a modern MICU, in a single room well-insulated for noise, becomes aware of the commotion that goes with the emergencies that occur with frequency on these units. Patients admitted to units with beds separated only by screens or curtains, live in the very midst of the crises that involve other patients. In addition, some patients experience one particular crisis—cardioversion for a ventricular arrythmia or cardiac arrest.

Druss and Kornfeld[16] carefully studied ten patients who had survived cardiac arrest. They found that not a single patient had faced the full implications of the arrest. All of the patients who had arrested used a variety of defense mechanisms (projection, displacement, isolation, denial) to control the anxiety aroused by the arrest and to avoid acknowledging its meanings. All the patients who arrested had frightening and violent dreams afterward. Hackett[3] also found that patients with arrest had frightening nightmares. Druss and Kornfeld observed hallucinations and delusions as sequelae to cardiac arrest.

At the present time, the best guide to nursing care following arrest seems to be the general one of understanding where the patient is in his effort to deal with an overwhelming psychological stress. It is clear that direct confrontation to break down defenses is not in the patient's best interests at that moment. The nurse must remain open to the patient, ready to talk about material with which the patient can deal. The nurse should also be able to relate some of the patient's symptoms of anxiety after the arrest in a general way to the event itself. The nurse is in the position to say, at appropriate moments, that she can understand the patient's being upset because of the difficult experience the patient has recently gone through.

Example: A 62-year-old man was admitted to a CCU with a myocardial infarction. Two days after admission, the patient experienced a cardiac arrest and was cardioverted. He was conscious at the time that the shock was administered. After he stabilized, the patient talked to a nurse about the experience. He reported dreaming that he was working on high-tension electrical lines and received a powerful shock from one of the wires. The patient's father was a high-tension line worker who was electrocuted while at work. The patient slept very poorly for the remaining time on the CCU. He did not report any other dreams.

Patients rarely indicate any wish to talk about or even acknowledge deaths of other patients. While patients are aware of the disruption in the unit when a major crisis occurs, the anxiety produced by such awareness acts as a deterrent to open discussion.

Example: A 48-year-old man with a myocardial infarction knew that a male friend of his was admitted to the same unit with a similar diagnosis a day after he was admitted. He talked to the nurses about his friend and asked about his condition. On the third day after the friend's admission, he arrested and died. The arrest team worked for over two hours before giving up. The original patient never mentioned this friend again for the remainder of his CCU stay, even though no one had told him that his friend had died.

It is difficult to detail specific nursing plans to deal with these situations because individual patient response is so variable. The one key organizer here is the nurse's ability to remain open to references to the critical event—that is, either observing another patient's death or the patient's own arrest and cardioversion. The ability to nurture and maintain patient confidence and trust will depend in part on the nurse's honesty in responding to the patient's questions about events like these. Careful explanation of cardioversion, when it occurs, could be done when the patient's condition is stabilized. For the patient who became aware of his friend's death but did not want to discuss it, sensitivity to cues that would permit a discussion could be important. Patients often "test" their nurses subtly about these matters and hope the nurse will pick up the clue that permits the difficult and emotion-laden topic to be broached openly. However, nurse intrusiveness by "forcing" a discussion in the cause of "honesty" is counterindicated for some patients, who may not be ready at that moment to deal directly with the feelings aroused by very frightening events.

Patients do show distress indirectly, as seen in the example of the patient who became angry on the day when there were several arrests and deaths on the MICU. This type of indirect expression of anger is actually quite typical. Observant nurses become aware that, on days following crises and on which several deaths have occurred, other patients on the unit will demonstrate more anxiety and other psychological symptoms.

Hackett[3] reported data on ten patients who observed fatal cardiac arrests. Seven of these patients denied any fear, either during or after. Three patients did admit they were afraid. The patients in Hackett's study distorted the sounds. Two of them were sure the chest had been opened and the heart massaged. Hackett, unfortunately, does not indicate whether emotional responses were demonstrated in other ways, as in the examples cited above.

DENIAL

There is general agreement that denial is a frequently observed and important coping mechanism, particularly in MI patients. Hackett[3] defines major denial as the unequivocal statement by the patient that no fear was experienced at any time during the hospital stay. Twenty of the 50 patients (40%) in his study fell into that category. An additional 26 (52%), identified as partial deniers, initially denied being frightened, but eventually admitted feeling some fear. Four patients (8%), who complained of anxiety or readily admitted to being frightened, were identified as minimal deniers. Hackett believes the major deniers habitually dealt with all emotional stress by repudiating it and that this choice of defense predated the MI. Twenty-eight of 45 patients admitted thinking of death while in the CCU, but only 11 of 42 admitted fear. Hackett sees major denial as having value for immediate survival. None of the major deniers died. Two minimal deniers and two partial deniers died during the study period, which was *only* the time the patient spent on the CCU. Hackett suggests a hands-off approach for major deniers, but active nursing care plans for partial deniers to reduce anxiety because these people want reassurance but do not know how to ask for it.

Hackett's data are more complex to interpret than his own discussion of them seems to indicate. Standardized interviews were not used and standardized psychological tests were not employed to validate the clinical descriptions of denial, anxiety, or depression. There is no information about the seriousness of the MI or complications developing during the CCU stay except for cardiac arrests and delerium. No physiological measures, such as urinary catecholamines, arrythmias, vital signs, or blood pressure, were used. Hackett's calculation of the number of deaths is confusing. Three patients arrested and died on the CCU. Another arrested and survived for 13 days in the hospital. Two more died within six months of discharge. The category of denial exhibited by these two patients is not stated. The total deaths were six, if the six-month follow-up time is used.

Size, location, and number of infarction—e.g., whether it was the first or second or third—are important in determining mortality outcome. Hackett suggests a relationship between major denial and survival and minimal denial and death. Another possibility would be to add size and location and number (seriousness) of the infarction to those relationships. The sickest patients were not included in this study, and the sample is skewed in favor of patients with less serious illness. Seriousness may be related to open anxiety and fearfulness. That is, sicker patients have more difficulty in maintaining denial as a useful defense. It could also be valuable to know if the deaths were due to primary or secondary electrical (conduction) instability. If they were secondary, then pump failure would be the underlying cause and psychological mechanisms would play a lesser role.

Hackett felt that the major deniers had life-long patterns of using this defense mechanism. His finding of 40% major deniers raises some interesting questions. Major denial does not, in this writer's experience, appear with such a high frequency in a general hospital population or in an out-patient population. Perhaps there is some relationship between being a major denier and developing a heart attack. Another possibility is that Hackett's sample is a rather special one.

What Hackett's data may reflect is that major denial is a useful and workable short-term defense as long as the illness is not serious. Major denial over the few days of an uncomplicated CCU stay could make it easier for the patient to rest, follow the treatment program, and begin gradual activity. Its value over the long haul might not be as great. If the denial resulted in disregard of treatment plans involving diet, smoking, and activity, it could lead to serious health consequences. In this regard, Wishnie[17] reported that 9 of 14 cigarette smokers in the sample went back to smoking within six months of discharge.

Dominian and Dobson's[18] study of 74 consecutive male admissions to a CCU underscores the points raised above. Three variables were found to be related to patient attitudes to the CCU: (1) social class; (2) severity of illness; and (3) patient perception of severity of illness. The lower two socio-economic groups, the patients medically evaluated as sickest, and patients who saw themselves as severely ill all found the CCU anxiety-provoking. None of the longer stay patients (over 8 days), the sickest group, found the CCU to be reassuring. Their data support the suggestions made previously that denial may work only in relatively uncomplicated, short-term cases. Miller and Rosenfeld[1] studied ten patients with MI in a CCU by using standardized clinical interviews and standardized psychological tests. They correlated these data with medications received, days post-MI, urinary cathecolamines, LHD, SGOT, and CPK levels, vital signs, blood pressure, and central venous pressure. They found an association between high epinephrine levels and denial. Miller and Rosenfeld believe that extreme forms of awareness control, such as a complete denial of illness, are rigid and ineffective coping mechanisms. They only appear to control the patient's anxiety while, in actuality, they aggravate it by generating conflict between patients and nursing staff.

Miller and Rosenfeld are not measuring the same variable as Hackett is. Hackett's patients admit to illness. They are deniers in that they do not admit into awareness the fear that would be a logical part of a life-threatening illness. Miller and Rosenfeld's patients "deny" they are ill and reject all information to the contrary. This mechanism is more accurately described as repression. Their findings are important ones for CCU staff to be aware of, but are not as helpful in understanding denial.

Gentry[2] studied denial on the CCU in 16 patients with MI. They used Hackett's definition of denial and thus examined the same variable. Gentry identified eight major deniers and eight nondeniers and studied them with standard interviews and standard psychological tests for five days. One important finding was that standard psychological tests could be used and that they provided objective measures, in addition to the clinical interview. Gentry found that deniers did not show any change in perceived current health status from Day 1 to Day 5 of their CCU stays, while nondeniers did. Only nondeniers demonstrated a decrease in anxiety during their CCU stays.

Nondeniers and deniers showed similar disruptions in cardiovascular activity (elevations in blood pressure). Nondeniers gained in feelings of security and assurance over time, while deniers did not change. In Gentry's sample as in Hackett's, the only deaths (two) in a six-month follow-up were patients who were nondeniers. Gentry does not say when the deaths took place or whether they were pump failure deaths or electrical instability deaths.

Gentry's work supports Hackett's findings. But, again, the seriousness of the MI and its relationship to the deaths in the sample is not clarified. But, because of this, until better studies are reported, it seems premature to say that there is a relationship between denial and death. The short-term utility of denial emerges in Gentry's work. But the nondeniers end their five days with an ability to more accurately appraise their physical condition. This raises the question of how denial and long-term survival are related. Hackett and Weisman's[12] study, which compared patients with MI and patients with terminal cancer, suggests that,when an illness moves from a short-term one with little pain and a good prognosis to a long-term, chronic one with much pain, a constant reminder of death, and a dismal prognosis, denial losses its value as an adaptive defensive mechanism.

There is a consensus that an efficiently working defense should not be challenged. However,this does not mean that the nurse should ignore the defense or whatever feelings and conflicts it is used to avoid. The nurse must remain open to the patient and ready to allow the patient to talk about concerns as they emerge. For some individuals, the denial may only be a transient phase in coping with the crisis of MI. Another reason for the nurse to be ready to assist the patient who is able to replace denial with more realistic coping maneuvers is that nonexpressive patients have been found to have high catecholamine levels.[19] Catecholamines are implicated in the production of arrhythmias, and reduction of excessive catecholamine secretion may improve electrical stability of the myocardium.

There is an additional perspective that may be used in sorting out the best therapeutic orientation toward the display of denial. Denial can be considered to have two separate components. One component is verbal and the other component is behavioral. One can divide patients who exhibit denial into four categories. In category one there are patients who displayed neither verbal nor behavioral denial. These patients acknowledge their illness and also behave in ways to maximize their chances of recovering and of protecting their health. The second category includes patients who exhibit verbal denial but whose behavior is characterized by efforts to follow the medical regimen and to protect their health. In both of these two categories of patients there would be little reason to be concerned about the use of denial.

The third category consists of patients whose verbal behavior does not exhibit denial but whose behavior does. These patients acknowledge anxiety about their illness, acknowledge that they understand the need for the medical regimen that has been prescribed, but behave in ways that are inconsistent with the medical regimen and, in fact, embark on behaviors that endanger their health rather than attempt to preserve it. The fourth category consists of patients who exhibit both verbal and behavioral denial. These patients do not acknowledge any evidence of concern or fear about their health and also behave in ways that indicate that they do not think they are ill. These patients not only deny any anxiety about their illness but also engage in behaviors that are potentially dangerous to them. It is with these two categories of patients that nursing staff should be most concerned. These situations call for contacts with the patient in open, nonjudgmental ways to try to help both the patient and the nurse understand the patient's need for, and use of, particular kinds of denying behaviors.

While no studies have been done to clarify these issues, it is this writer's opinion that the patients who exhibit denial in the hospital and who do well, both while they are on the ICU and in the postdischarge period, are predominantly patients in the first two groups described. That is, they are patients whose behavior is consistent with acknowledgment of the consequences of their illness. The corollary to this is that patients whose behavior, as well as verbal statements, exhibit denial tend in the long run to develop more complications. This is a hypothesis that needs to be examined closely and to be carefully tested in order to demonstrate its usefulness.

HIGH-RISK PATIENTS

The discussion in the preceding section on deaths among minimal deniers and the discussion in Chapter Four of the "giving-up—given-up" complex focused on two characteristics that appear to be related to poor prognosis for the MICU-CCU patient. There are other variables that have been identified as predictors of poor outcome, for the presence of which the nurse should be alert.

Rahe[20,21] discovered a relationship between a high number of recent life stresses, such as divorce, grief, and altered work patterns, and death from heart attack. Greene[22] reported that the majority of a series of 26 men who died suddenly of heart attack were depressed for a week to six months. In most of the cases, death occurred when there was a sudden arousal due to increased work or when circumstances produced feelings of anxiety or anger.

Obier[6] studied 57 patients in a CCU with MIs. Depression, pessimism, maladaptive family relationships, and poor social adaptation were significantly more common among those who died or responded poorly to rehabilitation. In this study, there was no difference between the psychological functioning of the survivors and the nonsurvivors during the CCU stay. In addition to the depression and pessimism, nonsurvivors continued to cling to past lifestyles and coping mechanisms and made unrealistic plans for employment.

Another variable related to poor outcome is the recent death of a husband or wife. Parkes[23] and Rees and Lutkins[24] both found that recent bereavement increased the likelihood of sudden death. In Parkes' study, during the first six months after the death of a wife, in 4,486 widowers, 55 years of age or older, there was a death rate 40% above the expected rate for married men matched for age.

In Rees' and Lutkins' study, widowers' death rates were about four times greater than married men matched for age. Widows also showed significantly higher death rates, but not as dramatically as did widowers.

From this sampling of the literature, a picture emerges of patients with a cluster of psychosocial characteristics that is related to a high risk of death. To recapitulate, these factors are: (1) depression; (2) sudden changes in life situations—especially those that lead to anxiety and anger; (3) recent bereavement, especially among men; and (4) pessimism or "giving up." Patients with these characteristics deserve special attention as soon as they are identified.

Their nursing care plans should include efforts to deal with the depression and hopelessness. They should also be considered for early referral for psychotherapy.

SUMMARY

Frequently seen symptoms in MICU and CCU patients are anxiety and depression. Both are amenable, in many instances, to appropriate nursing intervention. The sensitive nurse who makes the timely and accurate diagnosis can provide support, understanding, and treatment for patients with these symptoms. Anger and inappropriate sexual behavior are regularly seen in patients in MICUs and CCUs. Most often they represent maladaptive coping mechanisms on the patient's part, but they are complicating because they often are responded to with such strong feelings by nurses that problems arise in effective patient care. Patient deaths and transfers from the MICU and CCU are frequent sources of patients' stress and can be dealt with effectively by the nurse if she is adequately prepared to recognize them in advance.

Denial, often a mystifying or loosely interpreted term, is a major coping mechanism seen in MICU and CCU patients. It appears to be protective and related to good outcome with some patients. This may only be true, however, where the denial is primarily limited to verbal behavior and does not involve motor behaviors that are associated with an increasing risk of death from heart disease.

There are a number of factors associated with especially high death rates for patients on MICUs and CCUs. These primary factors are: high open levels of anxiety, hopelessness, and giving up; and a large number of recent life stresses, such as divorce, grief, and altered work pattern, and the recent death of a husband or wife. The MICU and CCU nurse can play an important role in promptly identifying these patients and taking part in their care by the institution of active treatment programs for the psychological distress demonstrated by these patients.

REFERENCES

1. Miller WB, Rosenfeld R: Psychophysiological Study of Denial Following Myocardial Infarction. J Psychosom Res 19: 43–54, 1975

2. Gentry WD, Foster S, Haney T: Denial as a Determinant of Anxiety and Perceived Health Status in the Coronary Care Unit. Psychosom Med 34: 39–44, 1972

3. Hackett TP, Cassem NH, Wishnie HA: The Coronary Care Unit—An Appraisal of Its Psychological Hazzards. NEJ Med 279: 1365–1370, 1972

4. Stern MJ, Wasail G, Pascale L, et al: Life Adjustment Post Myocardial Infarction: Determining Predictive Variables, Arch Int Med 137: 1680–1685, 1977

5. Kavanagh J, Shephard A: Depression After Myocardial Infarction. Can Med Assoc J 113: 23–27, 1975

6. Obier K, Haywood LJ, MacPherson M: Predictive Value of Psychosocial Profiles Following Acute M.I., J Na Med Assn 69: 54–61, 1977

7. Klein RF, Dean A, Wicson LM, et al: The Physician and Post Myocardial Infarction Invalidism. JAMA 194: 123–128, 1965

8. Gruen W: Effects of Brief Psychotherapy During Hospitalization Period on Recovery Process in Heart Attacks. J Consult Clin Psychol 43: 223–232, 1975

9. Parker DL, Hodges JR: Delerium in a Coronary Care Unit. JAMA 201: 132–133, 1967

10. Rowlett D, Dudley D, Early R: Emergency Use of Intravenous Haloperidol. Read at 131 Meeting of Am Psycho Assn, May 1978

11. Cassem NH, Sos J: Intravenous Use of Haloperiodol For Acute Delerium in Intensive Care. Read at 131 Meeting of Am Psych Assn, May 9, 1978

12. Hackett TP, Weisman AD: Denial as a Factor in Patients With Heart Disease and Cancer. Ann N Y Acad Sc 164: 802–817, 1969

13. Case RB, Millman HE: Psychiatric Aspects of Myocardial Infarction. Primary Cardiology 11: 15–20, 1978

14. Levy, NB: The Psychology and Care of the Maintenance Hemodialysis Patient. Heart and Lung 2: 400–405, 1973

15. Klein RF, Kliner VA, Zipes DP, et al: Transfer from A Coronary Care unit. Arch Int Med 122: 104–108, 1968

16. Druss RG, Kornfeld DS: The Survivors of Cardiac Arrest. JAMA 201: 75–80, 1967

17. Wishnie HA, Hackett TP, Cassem NH: Psychological Hazzards of Convalescence Following Myocardial Infarction. JAMA 215: 1292–1296, 1971

18. Dominian J, Dobson M: Study of Patients' Psychological Attitudes to a Coronary Care Unit. Br J Med J 4: 795–798, 1969

19. Klein R, Garrity J, Geline J: Emotional Adjustment and Catecholamine Excretion During Early Recovery From Myocardial Infarction. J Psychosom Res 18: 425–434, 1974

20. Rahe RH, Bennett L, Romo M, et al: Subjects' Recent Life Changes and Coronary Heart Disease in Finland. Am J Psych 130: 1222–1226, 1973

21. Rahe RH, Romo M, Bennett L, et al: Recent Life Changes, Myocardial Infarction and Sudden Death Studies in Helsinki. Arch Int Med 133: 221–228, 1974

22. Greene WA, Goldstein S, Moss AJ: Psycho-Social Aspects of Sudden Death. Arch Int Med 129: 725–731, 1972

23. Parkes CM, Benjamin B, Fitzgerald R: Broken Heart: Statistical Study of Increased Mortality Among Widowers. Br Med J 1: 740–743, 1969

24. Rees WD, Lutkins SG: Mortality of Bereavement. Br Med J 4: 13–16, 1967

CHAPTER 10

Psychological Aspects of MICU-CCU Nursing: The Nurses' View

Nathan M. Simon

Experienced MICU nurses were invited by the author on many occasions to talk about their emotional responses to ICU nursing practice. They shared a tremendous range of experience with much candor and openness—sometimes experiences that were painful or unpleasant to broach. What follows is a distillation and condensation of the emotional aspects of the experience of the MICU nursing practice of these nurses. The author has attempted to be as faithful as possible to the exact language and spirit of the information shared. Some of it may possibly be unique for a given nurse, but much appears to be generally true because so many of the experiences were echoed in separate sessions by different nurses.

ON BECOMING AN ICU NURSE

ICU nurses are both born and made. They are born in the sense that ICU work has become the new frontier and attracts competent, adventurous, assertive, competitive nurses. ICU nurses are made in the sense that there is a process of personal growth, learning, and testing that takes place before a firm identity is established.

ICU nurses generally report that the first three to six months of work are trying, arduous, and often anxiety-filled times. The nurses come to ICUs, their heads filled with a universe of new information, with untested skills, and impressed with the narrow margin of error their patients can tolerate. There is a nagging insecurity about what one knows, uncertainty about applying what has been learned, and a pervasive and haunting fear of doing something wrong. The new ICU nurse sees with awe the experienced ICU nurse working efficiently through crises, quickly analyzing and responding to emergencies, and setting treatment procedures into motion. The prayers of the new ICU nurse are variously "no arrests on my shift, please;" "May my patients have uncomplicated chemistries and gases;" "Keep the ventilator from fouling up;" "I hope nobody asks me a question I can't answer." The wish is to do what is expected and keep down the number of "obvious blunders." Guilt over not being completely and totally competent is an ever-present concern. At the same time, the new ICU nurse is tentatively applying new and not fully integrated skills. The exposure to frequent patient deaths and therapeutic stalemates add an element of discouragement and depression to this early period. Despite the intensive and sophisticated preparation new ICU nurses now receive in most hospitals, this initial period of uncertainty and complexity is still a real phenomenon. Some ICUs and CCUs have instituted a period of preceptorship for the beginning ICU nurse, which allows the development of competence and the sorting out of skills during a period of close work with more experienced colleagues.

The situation changes imperceptibly. The new nurse lives and works through cardiac arrests, identifies arrythmias, understands the chemistries, and survives the agonies of mistakes and of not knowing. There is growing confidence in clinical judgment, excitement and pleasure from performing well, and a feeling of the headiness of successful mastery. An important part of this phase is the participation in, and the ability to use, the mutual support system that nurses provide one another. The close teamwork required during even routine operation and the appreciation of a common, shared experience of hard work and stress lead to a willingness to reach out to help and comfort and to permit the acceptance of comforting when the pressures are the greatest. This support system contributes to the feeling of eliteness that begins to emerge. This eliteness is quite typical of small groups that work in somewhat isolated circumstances and are called on to do dangerous and special jobs. The feeling of eliteness contributes to some sense of superiority, which is an element in stabilizing the beginning ICU nurse as she takes on difficult and complicated nursing tasks.

The time arrives when confidence about one's judgment, skills, and techniques allows a reassessment. The new ICU nurse discovers that even more experienced colleagues do not know all the answers. A feeling of being on par with the experienced staff, and of even having moments of superiority, grows. There is often a reappraisal of what has been learned and a decision to learn more to correct perceived deficits. In this phase, there is sometimes a reawakening of the early anxiety that now is related to increased responsibility when the next "new" group of nurses arrives on the unit and the former beginners are now looked up to for guidance and expertise.

The next phase can be characterized as the "confident veteran." By now, the nurse has the feeling of having seen, heard, and lived through everything possible in the MICU-CCU—clinical and administrative. For some, there will be increases in responsibiities to Assistant or Head Nurse positions. The nurse will have ridden the rollercoaster of emotional highs and lows that is part of ICU work and will know the toll it takes in physical and emotional exhaustion that is often carried home. Periods of anger, discouragement, and pessimism are experienced, but are bounced back from with some resiliency.

For some nurses, this phase may conclude with a change in career directions. A significant number will move out of the ICU to positions—many times, leadership ones—on regular wards, in special labs, education departments, and nursing administration. Others will leave nursing to become mothers and homemakers. A few will find ways to replenish their depleted reserves and go back to the work that, for all its technical difficulty and pain, is the source of satisfaction and pride.

THE EMOTIONAL BRAIN DRAIN

The patients are ill—critically ill—and, when conscious, are frightened and needy. Their illnesses are often complex. There are cardiac arrests and other emergencies that occur regularly. The nursing care plans are intricate. There is never enough time. There is a demand for constant vigilance. The patient must be observed frequently and carefully for many parameters. There is a feeling of high performance expectation from the physicians and from nursing colleagues. There is an anxious family asking for information and support. The nurse must regularly struggle to understand and communicate with the patient whose capacity to communicate is impaired. There are constant requests and demands, both direct and indirect.

The description above is not overdrawn. It describes a situation in which the energy flow is overwhelmingly in one direction—from the nurse outward. To use an economic analogy—the ICU nurse is always underwriting and financing someone in a near or complete bankruptcy. It is not just the tension created by serious illness and complex tasks to be performed, but the experience of a constant one-way giving. The nurse has to balance off this drain on emotional resources with the sense of professionalism, support from colleagues, and satisfactions from intellectually, emotionally, and physically arduous work.

The direct gratification from patients' families is not to be counted on. So many of the cases have poor outcomes that the patient is unable to provide gratitude and the family is too involved in grief. The constant emotional drain that characterizes one-way relationships with patients surfaces in an oftentimes pervasive feeling of exhaustion and weariness, and may be one of the major factors that contributes to nurse turnover in MICUs.

IT'S NO FUN TO BE A LOSER

Death is a much more regular part of CCU and MICU nursing than in other parts of hospital nursing. The constant living with, and caring for, the dying and the families of the dying subject nurses to repetitive experiences of loss and to the reawakening of painful feelings related to personal losses. Death is frequently experienced by nurses as a defeat and as evidence of the failure of their skills. Professional identities are established and reinforced by successful application of skills. Frequent deaths challenge the establishment and maintenance of firm professional identity. Death confronts the nurse with the recognition of the limits of her science and art. Deaths uncover repetitively the core of helplessness that all of us have within us as part of human development. The nurse becomes aware that all professional skills have been used and that those skills have had no effect. It is "no fun to be a loser" and it is exquisitely painful to be reminded of one's helplessness.

Yet there are many times when the patient's death is accepted, welcomed, and even openly wished for. Acceptance of the patient's death or wish for a patient's death can develop when there has been a long period of mourning for the patient while the patient is still alive. It can also grow from the wish to see an unbearably painful situation resolved.

Example: The patient was a 74-year-old married man with end-stage COPD. He had several admissions to the same MICU over a period of three years. The current admission had gone on for eight weeks. The patient had been very popular with all the nursing staff, and the patient's wife had grown quite close to many of the nurses. There had been many arguments and very strong feelings because the nurses had felt that the patient should have been no-coded early in his hospital admission. For the last two weeks of his life, blood gases were constantly bad and there were cardiac complications.

The patient was finally no-coded and died within 36 hours. One nurse who had known him over the course of all his hospitalizations refused assignment to him on the day he was no-coded. She avoided the patient's wife and reported later that she felt just too depressed. She said the patient had spoken to her about dying a few days before and talked about wanting to go "asystole." Another nurse reported feeling sad for the wife. She felt the patient was peaceful because of his religious beliefs. Another nurse who had known the patient for his entire hospitalization cried for the patient on the days that he was no-coded and before he died. She spent as much time as she could with the patient's wife, having known her from the patient's first admission. She spoke with the patient's son about not leaving the wife alone. She had been assigned to the patient during one of the days he was no-coded and talked about making "social calls" into his room. She was in some ways surprised that the decision about no-coding did not produce a bigger response within her. Another nurse recalled her experience with the wife. The patient had been on a salt-free diet. The wife had asked why it was necessary to deny him salt when he was so close to death. The nurse felt extremely guilty. She was also uncomfortable when, as the patient's condition worsened and on the day of his death, she became aware that she did not want to come into the unit. Another nurse was aware of feeling very relieved. After the patient died, she sought out the wife, who was in the waiting room crying. She was aware that, in the last week of the patient's life, she had avoided the patient somewhat, even though she had made perfunctory visits to his room. She invited the wife into the nursing station where she and other nurses talked with her.

It is not only that MICU and CCU nurses must deal frequently with death, but that they are also, with great regularity, drawn into the "code-no-code problem." Decisions are made, and sometimes avoided, every day about the extent to which life-saving resuscitation efforts will be used on a given patient. Nurses are caught up in conflicts that grow out of this. Nurses find themselves angry and at odds with physicians about extended and repeated resuscitation efforts with patients who are thought to be terminal and without hope of recovery. Nurses sometimes find themselves divided about a decision to no-code a specific patient. Nurses will sometimes bitterly complain that a patient should be "no-coded." The nurses will be angry at the physician who fails to write the order to no-code. Yet, at the same time, the nurse may feel so guilty when the decision is made that even more anger will be directed at the physician who finally wrote the order. Nurses will often feel a sense of great injustice and resentment that one specific patient will be no-coded while another is not. The nurses feel that often there is little or no logic in the way decisions are made about no-coding patients. It is a frequent experience for the nurse to be caught up in the struggles that go on between physicians about the "no-code" matter. The patient's status may be changed from "code" to "no-code" and back again. At other times, there will be physician avoidance of responsibility about the decision that leaves the nurses feeling frustrated and resentful. Sometimes nurses are in the position of dealing with a physician who is unable to accept the impending death of a patient. All of these issues become sharpened and more poignant and difficult for nurses when the patient is young or with patients who are close to the age of the nurse's parents.

Example: The patient was a 70-year-old man with severe pulmonary edema, congestive heart failure, digitalis toxicity, COPD, chronic renal failure (BUN greater than 70), and CVA with the left hemiparesis. The patient was intubated on admission. He was alert and cooperative. There was great indecision among physicians about the treatment plan. There were two "no-code" orders written and rescinded. The patient was being treated with Nitroprusside and Dopamine. However, there were no blood levels of nitroprusside being determined, as was the usual procedure, nor were there blood gases being done. There were orders that the patient was to be bronchoscoped once a day. Some of the medical staff wanted the patient to have a tracheotomy, but the patient's private attending physician ruled this out. The nurses were furious and frustrated and felt helpless about the indecision among the physicians. They felt that the physicians should either decide to treat or not to treat the patient. Their anger was further complicated because the attending physician was telling the patient he was doing great at the time the patient was close to death. The nurses were in agreement that it would make sense to them if all medications were stopped. However, as the nurses talked more about the situation, their own guilt began to appear and they expressed feelings very much like the physicians who were unable to decide exactly what to do. They talked about the need to do everything. The patient finally expired before a decision about the tracheotomy was made.

Example: A 52-year-old male with acute leukemia was "no-coded." He was a married man with young children. He had only been on the unit a couple of days, but the staff had very much identified with his wife and family. At the same time, an 82-year-old woman with a COPD and congestive failure, who had been close to death a couple of times, remained coded and had been resuscitated on a couple of occasions. The staff was angry that the older patient was coded while the younger patient with leukemia was not.

Death has "come out of the closet." Kübler-Ross' work[1] has become the touchstone for many nurses since its appearance. This has been a mixed blessing. The work served to make discussion of death more open and it has made many more people willing to work more empathically with dying patients. However, the four stages described by Kübler-Ross are accepted uncritically by many. She created, in the minds of some, the expectation that all patients would, if they were to die "successfully," have to negotiate those stages in order.[2] Failure to do so was evidence of some weakness. More recent work[3] had indicated the individuality of coping mechanisms evoked by awareness of death and points more to the consistency of coping styles across the person's life, including its terminal phases. The MICU and CCU nurses, faced with frequent exposure to death, may opt to use the ritual of "stages of dying" in order to help protect themselves against the emotional drain that comes from working with dying patients. It is more difficult to deal with the individual, idiosyncratic behavior of a patient directly without the benefit of an intellectualized system to suppress one's own feelings.

DOCTORS ARE SOMETIMES ANOTHER DISEASE

There are a number of problems that grow out of the physician-nurse relationship on the MICU-CCU. On most MICU-CCUs that have full-time house staff and full-time senior staff, there is a close, sometimes very informal, working relationship between nurses and doctors. In some hospitals, nurses on other units are well aware and envious of this.

Some MICU and CCU have physician-staffing patterns that provide stress for the nurse. In units where there is no house staff, each physician is responsible for his own patients, and there is a simplified chain of command and decision-making process. In units with full-time senior staff and full-time house staff, the nurse often is in the middle of somewhat confused lines of authority. While the full-time staff may write the orders and institute the procedures, the private physician still sees the patient as his own. Also, serious differences of opinion will develop between house staff and private staff, especially over such things as "coding" or "no-coding" patients and the vigor with which certain therapeutic programs should be pursued. These differences of opinion create much insecurity and frustration for the nurse. They also provide opportunities for the nurse to project her own ambivalence about complicated matters onto other people.

Veteran MICU–CCU nurses are more experienced and knowledgeable about dealing with certain kinds of emergencies and clinical situations than most new house staff, especially at the beginning of the training year. Less experienced nurses feel uncomfortable at the time house staff changes because an important source of support is not available.

Example: At a meeting of nurses near the end of the training year there was a sudden appearance of complaints about house staff. The complaints ranged from the mistakes in judgment the house staff had made to the house staff's vagueness about orders to such a degree that the nurses had to push them to clarify orders. Finally, it emerged that the nurses were not thinking so much about the current house staff but about the *change* in house staff that was to occur in a few weeks. They talked about how they felt stressed because they had to act like doctors. While there was some pleasure in this and feelings of superiority, there was also discomfort and anxiety, and they talked about how difficult the first months of the training year were.

There is a competition present at times on MICU-CCU between the nurses and physicians. It develops from the special skills nurses have learned and mastered that many physicians see as *their* province of expertise. Junior house officers are most vulnerable and threatened by the expertness of the experienced MICU-CCU nurses. They sometimes respond aggressively and hostilely by asserting authority in nonfunctional ways. It's also true that the competitiveness is two-sided. That is, nurses at times get pleasure out of showing that they know more and are more competent than some physicians. In addition, house officers and attending physicians serve as displacement targets for strong feelings about other people who cannot be so conveniently attacked. Many times, attack on house officers serves the purpose of maintaining group cohesiveness among nurses or as a way of letting off steam about unsolvable clinical problems.

Example: The nurses complained bitterly at a meeting about the new house officer who talked to them like they were "little girls." The nurse who first voiced the complaint was an extremely competent and experienced nurse. The discussion that followed focused both on the new house staff and insecurity and also on the feeling of superiority that the nurses had, at times, to the new house staff.

There is sometimes a very special problem that develops in relationships with physicians that relates to sexual roles.

Example: The MICU nurses were very angry and critical of the two house officers who were assigned to the unit in the first rotation of the training year. Initially, in the discussion, neither house officer was identified and they were talked about in neuter terms. They were described as being somewhat incompetent, with one more anxious and one more authoritarian in style. It then emerged that both of the house officers were women. The usual kinds of tolerance for the problems of new house officers were notably lacking in this meeting, at first. Some of the nurses then talked about how boring it was "without any men back here." After that, the nurses were able to talk about another meaningful aspect of the situation. They wanted the two house officers to do very well because they were women. They had set higher standards for them than they did for the male house officers. They identified very much with them and were angrier and more upset with their mistakes. They wanted the house officers to do a good job for *all* the women on the unit. After this was discussed, there were more expressions of understanding about the interns and, while the nurses were still critical of some areas of their performance, virulence was missing from the criticism.

Physicians have problems with particular patients because of their emotional response in the same way that nurses do. Often the nurse gets caught up in a special problem that grows out of that.

Example: The nurses reported that the house officers were causing much trouble on a unit. They had trouble waking them up at night to examine patients, difficulty in getting them to pay attention to nurses' opinions about patients, and difficulty in getting them to write specific orders. The house staff would sometimes give verbal orders and would fail to write them. The nurses' anger increased. There were some direct confrontations between the nurses and the house officers until finally the nurses went over the house officers' heads to the Director of Unit, who reprimanded the house officers.

Example: On the first night on duty for a new intern, a nurse was having difficulty with a patient who had an MI and who had a Swan Ganz catheter in place. The patient became agitated every time the nurse left the room, even for the shortest period of time. The patient exhibited infantile behavior, cursed, tried to get out of bed, was exposing himself, and masturbating. The unit was rather short-staffed that night. The nurse went to the new intern to ask for some help in managing the patient. The intern walked away, saying "I'm not going to get upset." The nurse was furious. The resident arrived on the unit, saw that the nurse was having trouble, and went in to help her with the patient. As they were both getting the patient quieter and back into bed, the intern came into the room and asked, "What's going on?," appeared interested, and wanted to help. The resident later wrote orders that made management of the patient easier. Afterwards, the nurse reported her feelings. She could barely stand the obstreperous patient and she was absolutely unable to tolerate an unhelpful house officer. She had tears of rage in her eyes, she said, when the intern walked away from her. The nurse talked to other nurses after the incident who were supportive and her rage abated rather quickly.

Example: A nurse approached a house officer about a patient whom she perceived as extremely anxious. She felt the anxiety was not just a purely psychological problem and felt there was some change in the patient's physical condition. The house officer said he wouldn't see the patient and wanted to give the patient more Valium. The nurse, on her own, drew blood gases and later spoke to the resident, who examined the patient and found a change for the worse in the patient's physical condition.

Failure by the physician to communicate adequately to the nurse, especially about what has been told to patients, often gets the nurse in the MICU-CCU into difficulty. The nurse is often uncertain about how frankly she can talk to the patient because she does not know exactly what the patient's physicians have said to him. The critical issue, once the nurse has become aware of an uncertainty in what has been told the patient, is whether the nurse will be able to clarify the situation with the doctors involved. The ambivalence that the nurses feel at times about talking about patients may allow the nurse to "use" the uncertainty in what has been said to the patient as a way to avoid clarifying the issue. Sometimes it is an easier way out to be angry with doctors about what they may have said or not said to a patient than it is to talk to the doctor to clarify what the nurse's role is to be and then to actually be able to talk to the patient about the problem.

SPECIAL PATIENTS

There are special patients whose specialness may have little to do with their illness. Dealing with these patients and their families often creates problems for MICU-CCU nurses. Special patients are often patients who are known well by the nurses—people like staff physicians, staff nurses, family of staff, or the patients of some important staff physician.

Example: A very well-liked physician was admitted to the MICU for cardiac catheterization. After the catheterization, bypass surgery was planned. The morning of the surgery, the patient suddenly arrested and died. The response of the nursing staff was very strong. There was much guilt, depression, and feelings of inadequacy. The nurses felt that they had let everyone down. The nurses became targets for angry comments by nurses from other units of the hospital, which further increased their feelings of guilt.

Example: A 57-year-old man, who was the father of a physician on the hospital staff, was admitted to the MICU following a large MI. He developed pericarditis, possible cardiogenic shock, and septic shock. The patient's condition deteriorated rapidly. He developed GI bleeding. It was thought that he had infarcted his bowel and ascites developed. The patient died very suddenly with what was later determined to be a rupture of the left ventricle. During the time the patient was on the MICU, his son visited frequently, often at times that were not regular visiting hours. His appearances were often felt by the nurses to be intrusions. The nurses were never able to ask him to leave the room at times that they normally would have asked other family members to leave the room. The son came to the unit immediately after the patient died. He and the nurse who cared for the patient got into a discussion in the hallway about the patient's death. They used very technical language. The son expressed no emotion. The nurse became aware later that she would have never talked with the family of a patient who had just died in that way. She became aware that, because he was a physician, she felt under stress—something akin to examination anxiety—that interfered with her usual ability to be empathic, understanding, and emotionally supportive at the time of a death.

WHY DON'T PATIENTS BEHAVE LIKE PATIENTS?

MICU-CCU nurses bring to their work their expectations of how patients are supposed to behave. Patient roles are well-defined in any given culture. In our culture, patients are expected to want to get well, to participate in a process of cure, and to seek out and cooperate with experts who would help cure them. In return for assuming these responsibilities, the patients are allowed certain privileges. They are exempted from the usual social roles, allowed certain feelings and emotions that are in other circumstances proscribed, and finally are permitted to be cared for.[4] Our society does not usually hold the individual responsible for becoming ill with physical illness and believes that the person who assumes the ill role is deserving of care and entitled to it.

Most patients fill the sick role close to the expected way. However, there are many who do not. They neither seek nor accept care. The nurses can become angry with patients who do not meet role expectations. The anger may lead to punitive, authoritarian attempts to make the patients feel guilty about their lack of cooperation or to a withdrawal from the patient. When patients do not fill their expected role, it frequently uncovers an often ignored aspect of the nurse's role—the sanctioned use of power and controls. The awareness of the use of power can produce struggles between the nurse and patient and also great discomfort in some nurses, who find open acknowledgment of this a contradiction to the way they see themselves traditionally as comforting caretakers, not authoritarian enforcers.

Another source of difficulty related to role is the confusion between the sick role and the dying role. In the dying role it is expected that the patient: (1) remain alive; (2) arrange for orderly transfer of property and authority; (3) take advantage of the necessary supports for life and cooperate in their administration; (4) accept the curtailment of freedom and loss of privileges imposed by caretakers; (5) cooperate with caretakers; and (6) face death with some degree of courage.[4] In return, patients in a dying role are exempted from the usual social responsibilities, entitled to supportive care, and entitled to continued attention and respect until the end of their lives.

Example: A 42-year-old woman was hospitalized with a cardiomyopothy of unknown etiology. She was in intractable failure. Her physician and the house staff wanted the patient to go to a hospital in another state to undergo a heart transplant operation. Despite considerable pressure from physicians, the patient refused to do this. All medications were discontinued after the patient refused the transplant procedure. The house staff appeared angry with the patient and some of the nurses shared in this anger. Other nurses were angry because they thought withdrawal of all medication was precipitous. All of them identified the patient as young and felt very upset by that. The patient was alert during the time she was on the unit. This patient was able to tell one of the nurses that she felt deserted by the house staff and by the nursing staff. Another nurse, who was angry about the discontinuation of medication, contrasted this patient with an 83-year-old patient with "no lungs" who had been on a ventilator for a long time and whom the house staff would not "no-code."

Refusal to shift from seeing the patient as sick-curable to sick-dying can cause feelings of disappointment, anger, and resentment. The nurse experiences the patient as resisting curative efforts. Even when the nurse does accurately identify the patient as dying, many patients do not neatly fit into the role the society assigns. Quite the contrary, in order to survive with some identity, some patients will reject all or most of what the nurses (and society) expect. The wish to have a patient "dying nicely" or "bravely" or cooperatively is essentially a wish to make things comfortable for all of those who remain alive—family, nurses, and physicians. It is an attempt to reduce caretaker guilt and anxiety. It also serves to convert a completely personal, mostly indescribable, event into a ritual.

The stress of MICU nursing practice described in the preceding pages is mostly of a sort that, in the long run, can be dealt with by working through and understanding feelings aroused in the nurse. The sources of these stresses are built into the ICU and remain a constant part of it. The very ill patients, the high death rate, the intensity of emotional response by patients and their families, the idiosyncratic coping styles utilized by patients, regularly recurring problems with new house staff and with medical staff, and the physically exhausting work will always be there. In Chapter 6, attention was paid to educational administrative tactics that can help with stress reduction. These tactics and strategies are valuable and need implementation, for, while they are not "curative," they at least open reasonable avenues to make stress and tension reduction possible.

But the type of stress primarily described in this chapter requires something in addition. Both private and shared understanding of feelings become critical elements in the resolution of the emotional states aroused by the more chronic continuing stressful aspects of ICU practice. The sharing and airing of the problems play a central part in stress reduction. An open and responsive leadership, nursing and medical, who takes the time to listen seriously to colleagues, the types of groups described in Chapters 11 and 15, where nurses may freely talk without fear of reprisal about the uncertainties and frustrations of their experiences, a well-solidified sense of professional role, and personal maturity remain the primary modalities in helping the nurse cope with the emotional complexities of ICU practice.

SUMMARY

MICU nursing practice has built into it a number of rewards and stresses that become part of the nurse's life. Initiation into

ICU practice is difficult and fraught with anxieties but, as successes accumulate, the highly professional, competent MICU nurse emerges. However, the special stresses of high patient death rates, the constant care of patients who are critically ill and can return little to the nurses in the way of emotional gratification, and struggles between nurses and physicians and among physicians over status and competency issues take a steady toll in the form of personal distress and pain experienced by the nurse. Most nurses will eventually move to other areas of nursing practice. A few will remain and, despite the stress, will be able to continue to function at a high level.

REFERENCES

1. Kübler-Ross E: On Death and Dying, New York, The MacMillan Company, 1969

2. Kübler-Ross E: Death—The Final Stage of Growth, Englewood Cliffs, NJ, Prentice-Hall, Inc., 1975

3. Schneidman ES: Aspects of the Dying Process, Psych Ann 78: 25–40, 1977

4. Noyes R, Jr: The Dying Patient: Establish His Role to Improve Care. Psychosom 18: 42–46, 1977

CHAPTER **11**

The Coronary Pulmonary Surgical ICU: A Nursing Challenge

James H. Billings, Neal H. Cohen, and Mary Brian Kelber

INTRODUCTION

Cardiopulmonary Units (CPU) have developed to facilitate the care of postoperative cardiac and thoracic surgical patients. While it is obvious that nursing requirements differ for surgical and medical patients and that centralization of the cardiothoracic patients facilitates the care of these patients, a variety of specific CPU-related issues deserve special consideration.

Intensive care units are specialized wards with a limited number of beds in full view of a centralized nursing station. Attempts at ensuring patient privacy are made, but often unsuccessfully, due to the critical nature of the patient's illness and the care and attention the illness requires.[1] Elaborate monitors and alarm systems are in use at each bedside. In the case of the postoperative cardiothoracic patients, chest tubes connected to suction drainage bottles and mechanical ventilators are commonplace, adding not only to the already cluttered bedside, but also to the high noise level obvious to any observer.[2] In addition, large surgical dressings create a sense of distance, a psychological, if not physical, barrier between the patient and staff.

As is true of all critical care facilities, the CPU staff is abundant and diverse. The nurse-to-patient ratio is high; rarely are there more than two patients being cared for by a single nurse. The more critically ill patients have a 1-1 nurse-to-patient ratio. In addition, the CPU has a high ratio of physicians, respiratory therapists, physical therapists, social workers, etc., all contributing to the care, but also the confusion and congestion, of an already tense, stressful environment. The responsibility for creating order out of this chaos and ensuring the delivery of safe and effective care to this critically ill patient lies with the CPU nurse.[3]

THE CPU NURSE

The basic commitment that underlies *all* forms of nursing is the dedication to helping the ill person achieve or regain health, comfort, and freedom from pain.[4] To achieve this outcome with postoperative cardiac and thoracic surgical patients, the CPU nurse must possess a special blend of technical skills, human relations skills, and a constructive self-awareness.

The CPU nurse functions at an advanced level of clinical nursing. This generally requires a strong background in nursing practice and frequently previous general intensive care nursing experience before specializing in postsurgical cardiovascular and respiratory nursing.

The CPU nurse assumes primary responsibility for the care of one or two patients. She becomes expert at systematic patient assessment and continually makes data and intuition-based judgments on necessary treatment to promote the patient's adaptive response to physiological alteration. She must also continually monitor the patient's emotional needs, as the postoperative patient has undergone a traumatic experience in the psychological sense as well as the physical. By doing so, the responsibilities of a CPU nurse put her in a unique and vulnerable position. Because the nurse spends her shift in contact with critically ill patients, she becomes expert in the care of these patients. Therefore, in emergencies, the nurse is often called upon to assume decision-making responsibility for the postoperative patient in lieu of the surgeon, who is often not readily available because of other surgical responsibilities. This delegation of authority places the nurse in conflict with her training, which allows action only on the order of a physician. The role of the CPU nurse progresses beyond the traditional limitations of nursing responsibilities. The nurse may then have difficulty bowing to the orders of the physician, who, when available, wants to resume full responsibility. This is particularly difficult for the CPU nurse who has become more experienced than the physician in handling specific emergency situations.

The successful CPU nurse needs to develop a personal perspective that encourages confident, independent performance, when appropriate, and a personal wisdom that helps avoid a defensive, resentful response when the physician resumes direct control of patient care. In addition, the nurse must develop and maintain a sense of personal integrity, which makes critical self-evaluation a component of professional growth. A strong sense of self-confidence is critical for the CPU nurse, especially as her functioning tends to be independent.

In addition to strong clinical skills, good communication skills are essential. One of her responsibilities is integrating and orchestrating the participation of other health professionals in the treatment of her patients. These include physicians, respiratory therapists, physical therapists, and others. Good communication skills are also necessary with the patient's family. The CPU nurse is the most active and visible member of the patient's treatment team and it is not unusual for the nurse to be the primary source of information and support for the family. As a result of the level of individual skill and the range of responsibilities assumed by the CPU nurse, she often finds it difficult to admit that she does not have all the answers. She also finds it difficult to accept what she perceives as inappropriate or incorrect care by other nurses or physicians.

THE PATIENT

The patients who are cared for in the CPU include patients who have had surgery for cardiac disease, either valvular or coronary artery disease, pulmonary disease, or thoracic vascular diseases such as dissecting thoracic aortic aneurysm. A number of years ago, the common disease for which lung surgery was proposed was tuberculosis.

At the present time, the most common indication for surgery on the lung is tumor, either primary or metastatic. The majority of these patients do not have significant underlying disease that would interfere with survival in the postoperative period. On the other hand, patients undergoing lung surgery, who have emphysema or chronic bronchitis, can be expected to have complicated postoperative courses with prolonged ventilator dependence.[5] The patient with valvular heart disease has frequently been disabled by his disease for many years, and most have underlying myocardial dysfunction that is not reversible. Many patients with coronary artery disease have had a previous myocardial infarction or serious, recurrent ischemic heart disease and have been forced to alter their life styles as a result.

In each of these situations, surgical techniques, when appropriately implemented, can bring hope to individuals suffering from debilitating heart or lung disease. There is increasing evidence, however, that the long-range success of surgical intervention may depend more on the emotional characteristics and predisposition of the patient than on the surgery itself.

Kimball[6] identified four different preoperative psychological levels of adjustment by extensive interviewing with 54 adult patients on the day before open heart surgery. At follow-up (up to 15 months later), the "adjusted" group had an unremarkable postoperative period and an overall long-term improvement. The "symbiotic" group (people who had adjusted to their illness and utilized the secondary gains that provided) frequently experienced postoperative delirium with specific neurological manifestations. Hospitalization was often prolonged, and long-term response was unchanged or worse than preoperatively. The "anxious" group (people who tried to minimize signs and symptoms of illness, were uneasy about surgery, and unable to talk about it) acted in the early postoperative period as if they were afraid to move for fear of waking up and finding themselves dead or severely mutilated. They showed little affect and were passively cooperative. About a fourth of these patients died in surgery and there were a greater number of cardiac arrhythmias during the hospitalization. "Given up and given in" had the highest mortality and either no improvement or deterioration compared to their preoperative function.

Preoperative preparation of the patient by the CPU nurse is usually limited to giving the patient a tour of the CPU, acquainting the patient with what the postoperative experience may be like, and responding to questions and clarifying misconceptions that might contribute to postoperative complications.

PATIENT'S POSTOPERATIVE PSYCHOLOGICAL RESPONSE

The emotional or psychological issues to be addressed during this period are more specific. Kimball[6] reports that ". . . post-surgery delirium lasting up to 36 hours can be detected in some degree in all patients." Manifestations of this delirium range from distortions in the thinking process to hallucinations and paranoid ideation. This acute organic brain syndrome must be differentiated from the cardiac psychosis initially reported by Blachly and Starr[7] and described by Kornfeld[8] as psychotic symptomology, which slowly evolves after a lucid post-surgical interval of about 3-5 days. The patient is frequently disoriented in time, place, and person. Kornfeld[9] suggests that the severity of preoperative illness and length of time on the heart-lung machine increase the likelihood of cardiac psychosis developing.

In addition to the acute brain syndrome and the psychotic states just described, there are a number of other issues in the CPU experience that have an emotional impact on the patient. The hospital itself is generally a frightening place for the patient and his family. For them, nothing is routine and everything is potentially frightening, including such simple treatment measures as IPPB (intermittent positive pressure breathing) devices and intravenous fluids.

The CPU itself can be a terrifying place even if the patient had an orientation tour prior to surgery. The elaborate electronic gadgetry provides a different experience for the patient when he is hooked up to it. It's difficult for the patient not to think periodically about something going wrong with the machines, especially when a ventilator alarm sounds and the patient assumes the ventilator has failed, even though he has been told about the alarm. At times the staff forgets how terrifying the choking sensations can be with suctioning or the emotional impact of receiving a relaxant drug that is occasionally used to prevent dysynchrony with the ventilator. Even though the experience of depersonalization can be devastating, it's difficult for the patient not to withdraw into that defense when he undergoes the range of treatments that are nearly routine in the CPU. It is especially important in these circumstances that the CPU nurse remember that her patients are also people and need to be treated as such. For example, the superimposed needs of the patient with a tracheotomy must be met to avoid the "If I can't talk, I'm not here" syndrome.[10]

It is increasingly clear that the emotional needs of the CPU patient require the CPU nurse to be multitalented if she is to provide complete nursing care. One of the basic talents required is the ability to like and accept people as they are. The ability to create and sustain a caring relationship with an individual patient is likely to be the single most important variable in promoting a positive psychological response to the CPU experience. Each patient comes with different preoperative experiences, concerns, and fears. It doesn't matter that two individuals may have had the same operation performed by the same surgeon. Their responses to the surgery will in some way be different. It is easy for the CPU nurse to become a machine while caring for an unstable patient who is encased in machinery. A patient in this state, however, is particularly in need of personal warmth and support.

As important as emotional needs are, however, they are only one of the issues of concern for the CPU nurse in caring for a critically ill or terminally ill patient.

CARING FOR THE CRITICALLY ILL PATIENT

Those patients admitted to the CPU are critically ill in terms of their preoperative illness, surgical intervention, and postoperative condition. The CPU provides intensive surveillance and interventions.[13] Most of the surveillance is done by the nurse with the aid of monitors that efficiently detect life-threatening abnormalities. In addition, frequent portable x-ray studies and routine laboratory studies are performed. Most postoperative patients are mechanically ventilated and some patients in cardiogenic shock may require intra-arterial balloon pumping. The elaborate equipment, while helpful, often presents a psychological, if not physical, barrier to the staff caring for the patient. The monitors are obviously useful in evaluating physiological changes in the patient, but they cannot replace the clinical acumen of the nurse at the bedside. Consequently, the CPU nurse is the most critical element of this elaborate surveillance system. The details of caring for the critically ill patient are formidable, but the CPU nurse manages extremely well with the majority of patients who improve. The patient who becomes terminally ill presents a completely different set of situations for the nurse.

CARING FOR THE TERMINALLY ILL PATIENT

The CPU nurse, like most critical care nurses, accepts the intellectual, and sometimes impersonal, reality of death. She faces death more often than she would in a general medical setting and she is academically aware that death is a possible consequence to the complex surgical procedures undergone by the CPU patient. She is also aware that her newly admitted postsurgical patient is for some time close to death, and that any errors in management might be fatal. This awareness of death tends to be perceived through an exterior of professionalism that is developed through a constant exposure to the threat of death and frequent association with the reality of death. In most ways, this stance is essential for the nurse to continue to function in a highly stressed and emotionally demanding job. A strong emotional response to the death of a patient could well prevent the nurse from responding to her other patients with the skill and dispatch necessary to provide competent care or could render her unable to respond to the grief of the family of the terminal patient.

There are some occasions where a strong emotional response is difficult to avoid. As observed by Simon[14] and Hay and Oken,[15] some patients have unique impact on a nurse. This may be because of a strong sense of identity or association between the patient and some individual in the nurse's life, including the nurse herself. This association may be positive or negative. The power of its impact comes from its ability to penetrate the nurse's professional veneer and make the death experience a personal and painful one. A different, but equally difficult, association is described by Cassem[16] and concerns the anger and consequent guilt the critical care nurse experiences when she finds herself wishing that a troublesome or unpopular patient would die.

Observing that the CPU nurse generally avoids personal emotional response to the death of a patient does not imply that there is no response. The death of a patient is at times experienced as an assault on her professional skills and a threat to her self-esteem. Observing a mourning family or reading a card that says, "Thank you, you did all you could," provides little recompense for the time and energy the nurse spent on behalf of her patient. Dissatisfaction becomes worse when there is any possibility that physician or nurse error is associated with an unnecessary death.[15] The maintenance of self-respect and professional pride is extremely important to the CPU nurse and cannot be underestimated.

The availability of a variety of life support devices in the CPU presents a special set of death-related issues for the nurse. The relevant question is, if the patient can survive only if sustained on machines, how long should such devices be used? As Kornfeld[10] points out, these are legal, philosophical, and medical questions. The actual response to the question of how long the patient should be maintained through artificial means is sometimes arbitrary and unclear. The order to resuscitate, intubate, or "call a code" may be so diluted with other types of nonwritten or nonverbal messages that it's not unusual for the CPU nurse to feel responsible for determining what emergency measures are to be implemented.

In some ways, the most difficult task for the nurse with a dying patient is to be available to the patient for support and comfort. Constant attention to the dying patient is difficult. An enormous amount of determination and energy are required of the CPU nurse to resist the temptation to retreat into the machines or the endless details required to care for her patient's immediate physical needs. The patient's greatest need may well be the simple presence of a caring, attentive individual.

OTHER SOURCES OF NURSING STRESS IN THE CPU

There are certain other unavoidable interpersonal situations that make effective responses to the medical and psychological needs of the patient even more difficult. These interpersonal complications include how physicians relate to each other in the CPU and how this affects the nurse, how nurses relate to physicians and, perhaps more important, how the nurses relate to one another.

As mentioned earlier, there are frequently a large number of physicians from a variety of disciplines caring for the patient in the CPU. While this brings to the patient the expertise of a number of medical specialties, this diversity of physicians interacting with patients and nursing staff creates special problems. The postoperative care of the cardiothoracic surgical patient obviously requires attention by the surgeon. However, the surgeon is frequently unavailable to deal with a variety of situations that require prompt attention. The CPU nurse is usually the person available and responsible for making the necessary intervention. Many of these decisions are best made by physicians from other disciplines. While the consultation services of a variety of doctors are useful for the patient, "care by committee" can often be cumbersome, with decisions being reached too slowly in a clinical situation that requires immediate intervention. Ambiguity of responsibility creates anxiety for the patient and the nurse, neither of whom has a clear understanding of who is in charge and who coordinates the care of the patient. In this situation, the nurse caring for the patient feels compelled to assume a level of responsibility for decision-making without a specific charge or without being confident of physician support in her decisions.

The allocation of responsibility for the patient in the CPU has been handled in a variety of ways.[17] Some units have a director, usually a surgeon or anesthesiologist who assumes overall responsibility for patient care. In this type of unit, the staff has a clear understanding of who is in charge and whom to go to for clarification of ambiguous orders or resolution of conflict. One disadvantage of this setup is that the referring physician, as well as the surgeon who performed the surgical procedure, lose some of the responsibility for patient care. Generally, an administrative compromise is reached that provides for optimal patient care within the constraints of a given institution. Whatever the final administrative structure, it is essential that the CPU nurse have a clear understanding of who is in charge of the patient care and who makes the final decision.

Another source of potential compromise in patient care is the situation in which the nurse becomes entangled in the interpersonal physician-physician relationship. In the CPU, conflicting personalities and rivalries between specialties frequently come into full display. The CPU nurse must avoid being caught in the middle or assuming the arbitrator's role in physician conflict.

The other side of this dilemma is the alarming frequency with which the nursing staff perceives that physicians close ranks to protect the prerogatives of the medical profession or to cover up what nursing staff may identify as physician error. This, regretably, leaves the CPU nurse feeling as though she is the only one vulnerable to being caught "holding the bag." The unstated message perceived by the nurse is that mistakes are made by nurses, not doctors. The resentment and anger aroused in nursing by "physicians' brotherhood" behavior precipitates a "nursing sisterhood" response that can disrupt mutual respect and professional harmony.

The complex nursing-physician relationship is further aggravated by the reality that the job requires the CPU nurse to work independently much of the time. The adaptation to working in tense, and often life-threatening, circumstances requires the CPU nurse to possess a strong measure of self-confidence and a sometimes inflexible conviction that she can handle any emergency situation better than anyone else. As mentioned earlier, this is an area of potential conflict between the CPU nurse and the physician as well as a source of competition with other CPU nurses.

In the CPU, there tends to be an enormous internal and external expectation that the best possible decisions be made regarding patient care. Often there is an unwritten standard of professional competence with which the entire staff is expected to comply. In the instance of a physician error, if the working relationship between doctor and nurse is not based on mutual respect, a destructive experience is possible. This is especially apparent in teaching hospitals where the house officers have had less experience than the nurse in the care of the critically ill patient. Vulnerable professional egos, whether physicians or nurses, make good patient care more difficult.

From the CPU nurse's viewpoint, the ideal working relationship is characterized by mutual respect and collaboration. The physician and the nurse seek each other's opinion and participate together in the planning and decision-making process regarding patient care. CPUs in which such relationships exist presuppose a large measure of trust. This may mean that the CPU nurse's assessment of the patient's needs is sufficient for the doctor to initiate change in the patient's treatment. It is increasingly common practice for cardiovascular fellows and residents who staff CPUs to acknowledge the expertise of the nurse and to independently seek suggestions on therapy plans from an experienced CPU nurse. However, in those situations where there is physician resentment regarding the independent functioning or level of responsibility assumed by the CPU nurse or mistrust of the RN's assessment and decision-making capabilities, unit efficiency is frequently impaired. The physician who will not collaborate with the CPU nurse or heed her legitimate concerns is often quietly ostracized or "frozen out."

Another potential source of conflict between the physician and the nurse has to do with how the physician may deal with the loss of a patient. As Hay and Oken[15] report, "fatal outcome in a gravely ill patient . . . tends to stimulate feelings of frustration, self-doubt and guilt in their physicians." He may, for example, use projection and behave in a surly and querulous manner. He may bolster his self-esteem by becoming imperious and demanding that the nurses "wait on" him. He may also rely on avoidance as a way of distancing himself from his seeming failure as a lifesaver. On the other hand, ". . . compensatory overzealousness may occur. . . ." The physician may order apparently heroic, but frequently useless, gestures for the patient who is beyond help. This burdens and frustrates the nurse as she is diverted from other patients and their needs because of the doctor's ego. Being left alone to deal with the full burden of the family's grief is also an intensely frustrating experience for the CPU nurse. She, like the physician, is vulnerable to the agonies of guilt, frustration, and self-doubt. The nurse, unlike the physician, does not have the physical escape available to her that the physician has. The option of retreating even briefly to collect her thoughts is not generally available to the CPU nurse.

In some ways, the most complicated system of relationships in the CPU involves the nurses' relationships to one another. As previously discussed, the CPU nurse possesses an extremely high level of technical competence. Her self confidence and strong sense of professional pride enable her to work independently under extreme pressure and make life-saving decisions in an almost routine manner. A sense of doubt or hesitation can be fatal for her patient. A personal belief that she is the best at what she does becomes an essential component of her professionalism. It is not uncommon for her to believe that she is better at critical care than most doctors and usually better than any other nurse. While this personal belief is an element of her strength and adaptability, it is also a major area of vulnerability and can make her job more difficult.

The process of striving for superiority precipitates a competitive situation where the nurse's self-esteem is constantly at stake. In this atmosphere, nurses' rivalry often exists between critical care nurses and other nurses in the hospital. Cassem[16] has pointed out that critical care nurses, as a group, are viewed as ". . . prima donnas who are overrated and underworked," by nurses from medical-surgical units. Cassem goes on to describe the difficult situation of a noncritical care nurse floating on to the unit and feeling that she was perceived as a menace. Even worse are the feelings of anger and frustration of the CPU nurse who is forced to float onto a medical-surgical unit.

Competition, jealousy, and resentment may exist between critical care and noncritical care nurses, as well as between different critical care units within a hospital. Nowhere, however, is this competitiveness more destructive than when it exists within the CPU. Potential sources of support are neutralized, and peers become rivals.

The level of stress under which the nurse works makes human error difficult to avoid. When error does occur, she has nowhere to go, no one to talk to. Exposure of the error leads to fears of shame, anticipated condemnation, and loss of professional respect. This atmosphere increases the pressure and internal expectations for perfect performance to a level that can be nearly unbearable.

In addition to the myriad difficulties described, perhaps the most critical to the CPU nurse is the high probability that she is emotionally and professionally alone much of the time. The literature suggests a number of possible solutions for these potential problems. One of the most commonly mentioned possibilities is a support group orientated to the special needs of the critical care nurse.[10,14,15]

THE GROUP

One of us (JB) conducted a group for CPU nurses for nearly a year. That experience provided a considerable amount of insight into the very real difficulties, described above, experienced by the CPU nurse. The group developed in a manner similar to the 4 stages described by Simon.[14] The group was initially formal, although there was, in the first session, a candid acknowledgment that there were many problems, most of them interpersonal. There was a great deal of reluctance to discuss the conflicts because of the vague, generalized fear that things would explode and get even worse. As a result, the early group sessions were controlled discussions of issues that only rarely dealt with personal concern. This group also experienced Stage 2, a period of increasing tension and anxiety as the nurses gradually began to address pressing issues. During Stage 2, 6 of the 16 members dropped out. In Stage 3, the group began to struggle in earnest with the issue of trust; specifically, how much they could say and still avoid retaliation. Four more group members dropped out during this period. When Stage 4 was reached, there were only 6 regular members of the group left working together at a fairly high level of trust. The group continued to have difficulty at points of very sensitive and personal interaction, but improved enormously in this regard. The group decided to terminate when the group process became primarily psychotherapeutic. The notion of group psychotherapy itself was not objectionable, but the members of the group determined that this level of contact would possibly compromise recently improved working relationships.

A nucleus of interpersonal support was generated among the 6 active members by this experience. The long-term impact of this support system on the function of the unit remains to be seen. The group was perceived by the members as being a useful experience, providing an opportunity, as recognized by Hay and Oken,[15] to express some degree of their hostility, to hear that individual concerns about guilt, fear, and uncertainty were shared by others, and to construct functioning channels of communication among the group members. In addition, the group facilitated the identification of issues that they could do something about and those that they couldn't change. There was considerable discussion of the value of acting in concert with one another and the disadvantage of rugged individualism.

These are all positive contributions to improving personally stressful working conditions. There were a number of conflicts, however, that the group could not resolve. The group could do nothing about increasing the level of the nurse's authority to match her responsibility. It could do very little, except enhance effective communication, about the rage that comes from feeling infantilized by an attending physician or excluded from the treatment planning process. Finally, it could do little to dilute the frustration they experienced at how medical staff tended to handle issues of competence in critical care.

It is apparent that much needs to be done to maximize the efficient utilization of all the resources available in the CPU. It is also clear that success in this task depends on the effective and respectful collaboration of nursing and medical staff. If groups are to be utilized, it would be useful to have medical attending staff and house staff participate with the CPU nurse. As Kornfeld[10] suggests, it would be useful for the physician to understand the special stresses faced by the critical care nurse. Each CPU is different, the specific problems are different, and the personnel are different. Specific solutions are available only if the problems are jointly acknowledged and the solutions mutually determined.

SUMMARY

Cardiopulmonary Units have developed to facilitate the care of postoperative cardiac and thoracic surgical patients. Because of the unique nature of the CPU patient population, the CPU nurse must possess a special blend of technical skills, human relations skills, and a constructive self-awareness. The CPU nurse must deal with the preoperative and postoperative emotional needs of the patient in addition to his or her critical physical status. She or he must also develop an awareness of her/his personal response to the patient who is dying and the impact of that process on the patient's family. This awareness, while necesary to prevent a general retreat into the machines and the endless details of caring for the patient, is also a potential source of stress and pain. The CPU nurse must also deal with the ambiguity of responsibility for the patient's care because the CPU nurse is usually the person available. It is the nurse who frequently feels compelled to assume a level of responsibility and decision-making without a specific charge or without being confident of physician support in the nurse's decision. The potential for becoming entangled in physician-physician conflicts or feeling left "holding the bag" when physicians close ranks are also sources of stress that the CPU nurse must deal with at times. Another possible pitfall for the CPU nurse is the possibility of competition or rivalry among nurses. The level of competence, self-confidence, and professional pride that enables the CPU nurse to work independently under pressure makes the maintenance of self-esteem an ever-present issue. In this atmosphere, rivalry often exists, and the competition, jealousy, and resentment that can result tend to neutralize potential sources of peer support. When self-esteem requires a perfect performance and the level of stress that can exist as a result of any of these issues makes human error difficult to avoid, the situation is a potential pressure cooker for the CPU nurse. One useful resource for dealing with issues precipitated by a potentially difficult working situation is a peer support group that is oriented to the special needs of the CPU nurse.

REFERENCES

1. Margolis GJ: Postoperative Psychosis in the Intensive Care Unit. Comp Psych 8:227–232, 1967

2. Bentley S, Murphy F, Dudley H: Perceived Noise in Surgical Wards and in Intensive Care Areas: An Objective Analysis. Br Med J 2:1503–1506, 1977

3. Bilodeau CB: The Nurse and Her Reactions to Critical Care Nursing. Heart and Lung 2:358–363, 1973

4. Jourard SM: The Transparent Self, New York, D. Van Nostrand Co, 1971, p. 201

5. Milledge JS, Nunn JF: Criteria of Fitness for Anesthesia in Patients with Chronic Obstructive Lung Disease. Br Med J 3: 670–673, 1975

6. Kimball CP: Psychological Responses to the Experience of Open-Heart Surgery. Am J Psych 126:348–359, 1969

7. Blachly PH, Starr A: Post-Cardiotomy Delirium. Am J Psych 121:371–375, 1964

8. Kornfeld DS: Psychiatric View of the Intensive Care Unit. Br Med J 1:108–110, 1969

9. Kornfeld DS, Zimberg S, Malm JR: Psychiatric Complications of Open-Heart Surgery. N Engl J Med 273:287–292, 1965

10. Kornfeld DS: Psychiatric Considerations in the Intensive Care Unit. *In* Kinney JM, Bendixen HH, Powers SR (eds): Manual of Surgical Intensive Care American College of Surgeons, Philadelphia, W.B. Saunders, 1977

11. Sgroi S, Holland J, Mariot SJ: Psychological Reactions to Catastrophic Illness: A Comparison of Patients Treated in an Intensive Care Unit and a Medical Ward. Presented at annual meeting of Psychosomatic Society, Boston, March 1968

12. Klein RF, Kliner VS, Zipes DP, et al: Transfer from a Coronary Care Unit. Arch Int Med 122:104–108, 1968

13. Weil MH, Shubin H: Centralized Hospital Care for the Critically Ill. *In* Safar P (ed): Public Health Aspects of Critical Care Medicine and Anesthesiology, Philadelphia, F.A. Davis Co, 1974

14. Simon NM, Whiteley, S: Psychiatric Consultation and MICU Nurses: The Consultation Conference as a Working Group. Heart and Lung 6:497–504, 1977

15. Hay D, Oken D: The Psychological Stresses of Intensive Care Unit Nursing. Psych Med 34:109–118, 1972

16. Cassem NH: The Nurse in the Coronary Care Unit. *In* Gentry WD, Williams RB (eds): Psychological Aspects of Myocardial Infarction and Coronary Care, St. Louis, C.V. Mosely, 1975

17. Kinney JM, Bendixen HH: Administration and Operating Procedures. *In* Kinney JM, Bendixen HH, Powers SR (eds): Manual of Surgical Intensive Care American College of Surgeons, Phialadelphia, W.B. Saunders, 1977

18. Gentry WD, Foster SB, Froehling S: Psychologic Response to Situational Stress in Intensive and Non-Intensive Nursing. Heart and Lung 1:1426–1430, 1972

CHAPTER 12

Psychological Aspects of Nursing the Hemodialysis Patient

Norman B. Levy

In 1961, as a result of the invention of the silastic external shunt, a method was established by which hemodialysis could be given on a maintenance-of-life basis to patients without kidney function. At that time the theoretical work had been done and the necessary mechanical "hardware" had been in existence that would permit life on the kidney, but for the problem of blood access. This invention permitted access to the circulatory system without necessitating repeated venipunctures, which eventually obliterate the superficial vascular system of the extremities. With the problem of access surmounted, a new era opened in which thousands of people yearly in this country alone who would have died because of kidney failure could now be maintained by these artificial means.

The early days of delivery of this system of health care were truly pioneering ones, in which nursing staff shared with other professionals a sense of bold adventure into the unknown as well as a sense of guilt in participating in a service in which entry of the patient or refusal of entry essentially was equivalent to the determination as to whether that patient would live or die. It was not until 1973, when the Social Security Act was amended and Medicare payments made available to all those with end-stage renal disease regardless of age, that this lifesaving treatment became available in this country to virtually all who needed it.

As for behavioral issues, nurses were among the earliest of professionals active in making psychological observations of these patients. Among the earliest observations were those having to do with the acceptance or rejection of the shunt as an integral part of the self, the defense mechanisms used by patients in responding to the stresses of this procedure, the failure of these defenses, the issue of dependency/independency, and the phases of adaptation of these patients as they went from being untreated and at death's door to a new life on hemodialysis.

With the passage of time, the position of nurses on hemodialysis units has changed. In the past, they served in the traditional role as ancillary caretakers to physicians. However, in more recent years, the procedure of hemodialysis has been placed largely in the hands of nurses. Essentially, nurses tend to run hemodialysis centers by themselves, relying on physicians to deal with special problems and to do periodic reviews of their work. This increased responsibility has placed great pressure on the nurse as a care giver. Concerning the nurses' responsibility in the emotional adaptation of the patient, they are often helped by the social worker, whose presence is mandated by the terms of the implementation of the new Social Security law. Unfortunately, mandated presence does not necessarily produce an adequate presence of a behaviorally trained person. Often social workers are compelled to perform many functions that are secretarial, leaving inadequate time to care for the psychological problems of their patients. In addition, almost all of the social workers are medically, rather than psychiatrically, trained. Psychiatric services are also of varying help. There is a relative shortage of psychiatrists who are truly interested in the care of the physically sick. In addition, the consulting psychiatrist is frequently peripheral to the hemodialysis center, may not be attuned to the special medical and psychological problems of these patients, and may be unable because of lack of interest and/or time to fully tend to their needs.

In summary, by virtue of the progress that has been made, there is a wider availability of this procedure, a greater responsibility of the nurse in delivering this heroic health care, and a relative unavailability of people specifically trained in behavioral medicine to aid in caring for the psychological problems of these patients. It is, therefore, important that nurses recognize the special psychological stresses of this procedure and the psychological complications so that they may aid in the early diagnosis and treatment of these patients. In addition, adequate knowledge may be used in a preventive manner, so that the psychological complications of some of these patients may be avoided.

The purpose of this chapter is to discuss the stresses of hemodialysis, the major complications, and what may be done preventively or therapeutically to help the nurse in the care of these patients.

THE STRESSES OF HEMODIALYSIS

The Procedure

Although medical complications do not commonly occur during the procedure of hemodialysis, they do occur occasionally. Alarms frequently go off, at times falsely warning of a disaster that will not occur. Air does get into the system, tubings do disengage and cause a loss of blood, patients do go into shock, and, on occasion, patients die because of a stroke or other effects of mishaps. However well the mechanism may work, the continual flow of blood outside an individual's body into a complicated set of machinery is never perceived as danger-free and, for most, constitutes an important stress because it is such an "unnatural" event. Intrapsychically, the exit of blood is connected with a major body mishap, usually injury and danger. The stress of the procedure itself is often reflected by the presence of insomnia in hemodialysis units. Masturbation is also a relatively common phenomenon in these units. Its presence is probably a method the patient uses to cope with anxiety—by using a sexual outlet—rather than due to any sexual problem, much like men about to face battle, who have also been observed to masturbate relatively openly.

The relationship of the patient to the machine is clearly an ambivalent one. It is perceived, especially in early phases of treatment, as a life-saving and life-protecting "friend." However, it also represents the life-long obligation of the patient to the procedure and is tangible evidence of the lack of health and of impaired longevity. Patients often refer to the machine as the "monster," or, at times, as "mother."

Dependency/Independency Conflicts

In no procedure since the external artificial respirator for bulbar polimyelitis have so many individuals been so dependent upon a procedure, a machine, and a limited number of personnel. The response of patients to this factor depends greatly upon their ability to tolerate greater dependency and, thus, upon their personality type prior to the onset of their illness. The very independent patient—that is, the patient who protests his or her independence—may run into major difficulties because his personality runs counter to his medical needs. Such patients may respond with anxiety, depression, and/or may use denial—an unconscious mechanism in which anxiety is kept in bounds by removing awareness of an external reality. This denial serves as a method of minimizing the impact of the necessity of this procedure and may result in the patient's setting aside his medical needs, resulting in his failure to adhere to the medical regimen or, at times, even to come for a scheduled hemodialysis. At the other end of the spectrum, the very dependent patient may find the situation of regression caused by illness and its treatment to be a gratification of his dependency needs. Such a patient may "enjoy" his illness and treatment and find that both occupy his entire life. Such patients become most difficult to rehabilitate because gratification becomes attached to the new dependency. The patient who can tolerate dependency and yet maintain as independent a course as is feasible often does the best. Such a patient is usually better able to handle the realities of medical and surgical illness while utilizing his independence as constructively as possible.

Stress of the Overall Medical Regimen

All patients with chronic illnesses yearn for some freedom from their state of having to be reminded that they are different from others. All but the patient with continual pain can gratify this wish. Respite from reminder of illness is an important part of adaptation to chronic disease and it requires the patient to utilize the defense mechanism of denial which, if used without interfering with the medical regimen, is usually a normal coping maneuver. The patient undergoing hemodialysis is at a distinct disadvantage compared to most others with chronic illness in that he is continually reminded of his illness and treatment because of the very nature of the treatment. The fact that this treatment is both lifesaving and continual places patients in almost constant reminder that they are different from what they once were and different from their fellows.

The author of this chapter interviewed 18 patients who had their arteriovenous shunt replaced by a fistula, enabling each patient to contrast for himself the two avenues of access to circulation.[1] It was discovered that all but one patient preferred the fistula to the shunt. However, the reason for the preference was not primarily a lessening of the danger of exsanguination, but rather of no longer having to have a bandaged extremity, necessitated by the shunt. A patient, expressing a view shared by most of the others, said, "With a shunt, I was bandaged and I was different and always reminded of being different from other people. Now I'm not branded anymore."

For all patients, the restriction on diet and especially on fluid intake poses great stress upon them. As in the case of other situations, the degree of stress is determined greatly by the type of person. Those with greater need for oral gratification and greater difficulty in tolerating frustration experience more stress than those with fewer problems in these areas.

The Stress of Unrealistic Expectations

Professional staff working in hemodialysis centers are usually exceptional people in many ways. They are usually individuals with professional accomplishments, who have chosen work that is very demanding upon them. As a group, hemodialysis professional staff tend to put on to others, including the patients for whom they care, their own high accomplishments. This is augmented by the medical model of rehabilitation as an ideal, with return to work and resumption of usual premorbid activity as a goal of virtually all health care professionals. Since patients experiencing the early phases of hemodialysis often have a relative euphoria, which has been termed as being part of the "honeymoon phase" of adaptation to this procedure,[2] the ground is there upon which unrealistic expectations may be planted. With the patient feeling optimistic, with the professional staff hoping that he will be able to resume his full previous activity, and with family hoping that he will be returned to active work, expectations for work, household, or school activity may be arrived at which may not be in concert with past performance, the impact of illness, and the realities of the new therapy. It is our experience that, if unrealistic expectations for productivity have been established, such patients may run into major physical and emotional difficulties when presented with a disparity between these expectations for activity and their failure to be carried out. In such a setting, we observed frequent medical complications and feelings of helplessness.[2]

The following is an example of such a patient.

"A 30-year-old carpenter, for the first time since starting hemodialysis therapy, was to subcontract for a major carpentry job. A few hours before his appointment, his shunt clotted irreversibly. Asked how he felt about the job, he said: 'I didn't know whether I could do it . . . I felt down in the dumps . . . I was willing to try . . . You never know until you try . . . I'll have to try again.' He also felt that the physicians at the hemodialysis unit would strongly disapprove of him if he had not reestablished himself as a carpenter. The patient continued to be discouraged and depressed and to have major shunt difficulties for several months. In the three years since then, he has never returned to carpentry and has worked only intermittently as a bartender."[2]

The Stress of Physical Illness Itself

Patients on hemodialysis enjoy a much better state of health than they did while they were uremic and untreated. However, they are never the way they were physically prior to their illness and usually contrast very strongly with others around them. No hemodialysis patient can resume the degree of activity that he had prior to his illness. In the words of the physician writing about his own hemodialysis treatment, "I cannot remember the last time that I can honestly say that I felt really fit. There are definite limitations imposed upon me, either by treatment itself, or the state of my health. I cannot function as well as I would like to. My fatigue threshold, although not as low as that of some other hemodialysis patients, is lower than I would wish."[3] Many factors cause this: They are chronically and severely anemic and intermittently uremic. They generally have complications of their illness and its treatment, which include secondary hyperparathyroidism. The additional blood flow caused by the fistula places additional stress upon their hearts, they have metabolic derangement, and generally a disequilibrium syndrome as a consequence of, and immediately after, the hemodialysis procedure.

The stresses of being physically ill are many and include the stresses connected with the many losses that these patients sustain. Patients undergoing hemodialysis have usually had either the loss of their job or a major compromise in their work productivity. This usually involves the stress connected with a lowering of income. There is loss of freedom by the very nature of their treatment. There is loss of strength, usually a loss in sexual functioning, and loss in their life expectancy.

PSYCHOLOGICAL COMPLICATIONS OF HEMODIALYSIS

Depression

Depression, which is a mood, affect, and/or syndrome, is the most common psychological complication of hemodialysis[4] and is a psychological response to a threatened, fantasized, or actual loss. For the many reasons previously stated, these patients as a group have many losses and thus sustain a fair degree of depression. There have been a number of reports concerning the origin of depression in these patients. One attributes it to a response to the failure of denial[5] and another to a response to being terminally ill.[6] One group, reporting on their 21 patients, rated one as being always depressed, one frequently depressed, 8 occasionally depressed, 6 rarely depressed, and 5 never depressed.[7] We found that, in 18 of the 25 patients we studied, depression preceded the onset of uremia.[2] In all 25 of these patients, depression was also clearly evident at the time of their acceptance into our hemodialysis program, when they were literally at death's door. With treatment by hemodialysis, we saw depression again at the time in which patients prepared to, or actually entered into, returning to work, school, or household activities. At that time there were distinct changes in their affective state, in which the previous feelings of contentment, confidence, and hope, which marked what we termed the "honeymoon" period, were replaced by sadness and helplessness. We termed this latter phase the period of disenchantment and discouragement, which we observed to occur gradually in some and abruptly in others and which lasted for about three to twelve months.

Suicidal Behavior

With depression the most common psychological complication of hemodialysis, it should not be surprising to learn that suicide is also relatively common among these patients. Unfortunately, the data on suicide are virtually restricted to a single study by Abram and his group.[8] This was conducted by a questionnaire sent out to 201 hemodialysis centers in the U.S. Of 127 returned questionnaires, the data concerned 3,478 living or dead patients. It was reported that 20 of these patients had committed suicide, 17 had attempted it unsuccessfully, and 22 had died due to voluntary withdrawal from hemodialysis programs. An additional 117 deaths were attributed to failure to follow treatment regimens. Unfortunately, there is a dearth of data on suicide in other groups of patients, making statistical comparison impossible. However, there are statistics on suicide covering the general population: 10 suicides per 100,000 in this country. If one uses these data to contrast the 20 successful suicides in the 3,478 patients, this would essentially mean that the prevalence of suicide was 100 times (10,000 %) that of the national population. If the additional 117 deaths attributed to failure to follow treatment regimen were considered suicides, this would increase the comparison to about 400 (40,000 %) times that of the general population. However, the national statistics on suicide are much lower than the reality of suicide for obvious reasons and, because of this, Abram's group has modified its statements about its prevalence and prefers that the suicide rate be considered many times that of the general population, rather than 100 or 400 times greater. Some investigators feel that the suicide rate of patients on hemodialysis is no greater than in other groups of seriously ill patients.[9]

The entire issue of voluntary control for programs of hemodialysis needs to be considered in the context of the issue of suicide. Although reality considerations may at times play an important role in a practical decision to withdraw from such program, it is the personal feeling of the author of this chapter that this is a relatively uncommon phenomenon. Voluntary withdrawal usually occurs when the patient gives up efforts to cope with the physical and psychological stresses of this procedure. Unfortunately, when such decisions are arrived at, they tend to be irreversible. McKegney suggests that the issue of withdrawal be taken up prior to the patient's starting hemodialysis, so that it may be discussed soon after serious consideration by the patient.[10] It is important that the hemodialysis professional staff carefully monitor the problems of psychological adaptation of these patients, including the presence of depression, so that issues concerning maladaptation, such as suicide, can be discussed early, and intervention, when feasible, recommended.

Sexual Problems

Initially, the major focus of hemodialysis was saving lives. However, with the mastery of technical issues and improvement of the hemodialysis procedure, there has been increased interest in the quality of life of these patients. Sexual functioning is an aspect of, and measure of, life's quality. Thus, satisfaction on the job, at school, or at home may affect the quality or frequency of sexual intimacy. If a person has problems with sexual dysfunction, it may be a reflection of general psychological maladjustment expressed sexually. If sexual dysfunction stems from physical reasons, it will tend to diminish the quality of life and it will place pressure upon the marital dyad to adjust to this loss.

In the years prior to 1972, there were no systematic studies of the sexual functioning of patients with end-stage renal disease. However, the observation was made that patients on hemodialysis seemed to have a considerable number of sexual problems. The one most clearly discerned was impotence. As is often the case in the area of sexual dysfunction, early examination of the problem ignored women entirely. In 1972, at a panel devoted to the psychological adaptation of patients on hemodialysis at the annual meeting of the American Psychiatric Association, Scribner concluded, "No data on this are good, but about one-third report that they are quite normal, about one-third say they have decreased potency but have some sexual activity, and about one-third reported they are completely impotent."[12] Since 1973, there have been several studies of sexual functions of patients maintained by hemodialysis and recipients of renal transplantations. The data clearly pointed the direction of major sexual dysfunctions in members of both sexes on both methods of treatment.

Abram and his associates studied, by semistructured interviews, the sexual function of 32 male patients maintained by hemodialysis.[13] The average frequency of sexual intercourse per month was found to be 10.4 before the onset of uremia, 5.7 after the onset of uremia and before hemodialysis, and 4.0 while maintained by hemodialysis. Fourteen patients had impotence after becoming uremic and an additional 11 after being on a hemodialysis program. Only 7 patients had no decrease in sexual function either after the onset of uremia or while on hemodialysis. Thus, 25 (78%) of the 32 patients had problems with impotence while being treated by hemodialysis.

The author of this chapter investigated sexual functions of maintenance hemodialysis and transplant patients by sending questionnaires to the 1,166 members of the National Association of Patients on Hemodialysis and Transplantation.[14] With a 67% response, the data were reported on 429 adult hemodialysis patients. They were questioned concerning sexual functions prior to the onset of uremia, while uremic and untreated, and after being treated by hemodialysis or transplantation. The measures of sexual function were: frequency of sexual intercourse in members of both sexes; in the men, prevalence of impotence; and in the women, prevalence of orgasm during sexual intercourse. The data showed a marked deterioration in sexual function in both sexes when the period prior to the onset of uremia was compared with that on hemodialysis. The number of men never having sexual intercourse increased from 27 before uremia to 135 while on hemodialysis. In women, they were 13 and 47, respectively, and their frequency of orgasm during sexual intercourse had also diminished since being on hemodialysis. Fifty-nine percent of the men reported that they had problems with impotence since being on hemodialysis. In this study, impotence was defined as difficulty in getting or maintaining an erection for sexual intercourse. However, 23 patients reported that they were "not sure" that they had a problem and 89 that they had "no problem." In analyzing the other answers made by these 112 patients, 42 stated that they never have intercourse at all now. The inference is that the true incidence of impotence is probably in excess of 70%

Initiation and continuation of hemodialysis was associated with worsening of sexual functioning in 35% of the men and 25% of the women. Only 9% of the men and 6% of the women experienced improvement in sexual function while on hemodialysis. Thus, in the situation of improvement in every other area of physical activity, a large number of patients experienced worsening of sexual activity. These data corroborate the previously mentioned study of Abram, which also showed a deterioration in sexual functioning as patients went from being uremic and untreated to being treated by hemodialysis.[13]

We see these latter data as indicating a likelihood of a psychological component in these sexual dysfunctions.

Much remains to be learned about the cause of the sexual dysfunctions. Certainly organic factors must play an important role in these problems. The patients are chronically anemic and intermittently uremic in addition to having other medical complications. Hyperparathyroidism has been incriminated.[14] However, more definitive work in this area still remains to be done. An additional factor is the antihypertension medication taken by many of these patients. Most of these medicines have a side effect that includes reduction of libido and they may cause impotence. Psychological factors probably also play a significant role. As previously mentioned, depression is a common complication, in which diminished sexual interest and ability is often a somatic concomitant. Other factors that could cause sexual dysfunction include the frequent reversal of family role, especially in male patients. Men have end-stage renal disease twice as commonly as women; most commonly they do not resume their work activity and often choose to be deemed permanently disabled. With reduction of family income because of their receiving disability payments rather than wages, their wives are often forced to enter or re-enter the work market. The absence of the wife from the home usually necessitates the husband's greater activity in household matters, which may include his cleaning, shopping, cooking, and caring for the children. Another factor of importance, primarily for men, is the cessation of urination, which stops that function for which the penis is by far most commonly used. The differentiation between the two functions of the penis is fused in the preconscious, so that the loss of urination tends to be perceived by the male patient, in varying degrees, as a castration equivalent. As in the case of reversal of family role, cessation of urination will affect a man to a degree dependent upon the confidence that he has in his own masculinity. Those of more tenuous masculine identity will be more affected than those in whom masculinity is better established.

Uncooperativeness

The lack of patient cooperativeness is among the major problems confronting hemodialysis nursing personnel. The definition of what is a "cooperative" and an "uncooperative" patient often has more to do with the needs of professional personnel than the realities of patients. The more docile and compliant patient tends to be seen as "cooperative" and the complaining patient, at times irrespective of cause or justification, tends to be viewed as "uncooperative." These factors are accentuated in busy services dealing with life-sustaining processes such as hemodialysis.

As previously mentioned, the patient who protests his independence may use denial in a manner that may interfere with his adherence to diet and other aspects of his medical regimen, resulting in the missing of dialysis runs. In such a patient, the personality trait of independence runs directly counter to medical needs. At times, such patients are advised to be transplanted because of their inability to tolerate the dependency demands of hemodialysis.

Perhaps the most common "uncooperative" behavior in hemodialysis units is the exaggerated response that patients occasionally have to rather minor mishaps. When there is a disparity between the actuality of the mishap and the response of the patient, one should think of the possibility of another factor playing a part—anger at their sick role. Although most patients initially are very grateful for being resurrected from either being near-dead or from approaching near-death due to uremia and then being resuscitated to the living on hemodialysis, gratitude soon gives way. Most patients are most affected by the fact that they are different from the way they once were and different from their fellow human beings. Often their response to their illness includes that of anger, which may become displaced to their available caretakers. It is important that the caring professional, especially the nurse who is often the primary focus of this displaced anger, not react in kind, thus adding credence to the fantasy of patients that they are not being cared for adequately. For example, a 25-year old woman entered a hemodialysis center with a pastrami sandwich and announced to all in the unit that she intended to eat that sandwich while being dialyzed. This occurred at a time in which the dietary restriction of hemodialysis patients was particularly rigid. The nurse on duty approached the patient and essentially gave her a choice between having the pastrami sandwich or receiving hemodialysis that evening, but not both. After a good deal of fussing and cursing, the patient sacrificed her sandwich in favor of treatment. After some time had passed and the patient was relatively comfortable, the nurse approached her and asked her how things were going. The patient complained that her boyfriend of many years had decided the night before to tell her that he wanted to break up with her. He said that he had learned that hemodialysis patients are bad medical risks and anyway that they can't have children. The response of the nurse in not being provoked by this "uncooperative" behavior, insisting upon adherence to unit policy, and successfully uncovering the source of the behavior was most constructive to the patient, her fellow patients, and to the unit.

Patient Rehabilitation

The entire area of rehabilitation of patients on hemodialysis is rather confused by varying definitions of the word "rehabilitation." For most people, that term refers to the return of people to the usual work that they did prior to their illness. The overwhelming majority of men, perhaps over two-thirds, cannot return to full-time work activity and essentially retire from the work that they had once done. A factor affecting patient rehabilitation is the nature of the very work performed. To some degree, rehabilitation is a function of the patient's hematocrit. That is, a patient who is a ditch digger is going to have much greater difficulty returning to that work than is a college professor. Furthermore, those occupations that are manual and physically strenuous are usually less flexible. Thus the college professor has another advantage in the opportunity he usually has to change hours according to his medical needs. These factors are among those explaining why patients of low socioeconomic position have greater difficulty in rehabilitation than those of higher status.[16] In addition, women tend to have less difficulty on hemodialysis than men. One factor of importance explaining this is that women still have greater options than men concerning employment in outside work activity. Women can still choose to do housework, which is more flexible and usually less physically demanding than most other outside work activities.

PSYCHOLOGICAL STRESSES OF NURSING HEMODIALYSIS PATIENTS

The long-term relationship between nurse and patient poses special stresses for the dialysis unit nurse. There is more opportunity for the patient to develop transference-like reactions (seeing the nurse with an emotional set appropriate to some important figure from early life) and for the nurse, in response to it to develop countertransference-like reactions to the patients.[17] The nurse must be prepared to deal with her own responses to frequent displays of anger, uncooperativeness, negativism, and depression. The nurse must also cope with a subgroup of angry patients who deal with the humiliation and mortification engendered by their illness by personifying their problems, displacing them on to the nurse, and then reacting with "justified anger."[18]

This long-term nurse/patient relationship also enmeshes the nurses more intimately into their patients' lives. The death of a patient may become a very personal experience and may not be dealt with as adequately by the usual distancing of the professional role. The intimate long-term relation makes patients more sensitive to the nurses' absences. Vacations or unexpected absences often produce depression in patients and anger that may be directed at the nurse on her return. This may often surprise the nurse who, instead of finding patients glad to see her back, may discover that they are angry, sulking, and/or creating situations that punish the nurse for the "abandonment."[19]

Sexual issues that are associated with this treatment pose a special problem for some hemodialysis unit nurses. Masturbation that is frequent and that many times is performed relatively openly can be a source of upset to the nurse. Care must be exercised to avoid punitive reactions that will isolate the patient, increase guilt and shame, and ultimately compromise effective communication.

Depression is ubiquitous among the patients and this usually has a personal effect on the nurse. Working with chronically depressed patients is often experienced consciously or unconsciously as a burden. The problem of depression is complicated by the high frequency of suicide that causes repeated and transient intrusions of guilt and anger into the life of the nurse who, like all members of the therapeutic team, inevitably feels a sense of responsibility when this occurs.

Kaplan De-Nour[20,21] and her colleagues in Israel have studied the attitudes and psychological responses of nurses who work on hemodialysis units. Because of culture differences, caution must be used in applying her data to other settings. But her findings describe important phenomena of general interest and deserve discussion. They found that the nurses frequently had difficulty managing feelings related to their belief that they had "given life to people who would otherwise be dead." The nurses expected the patients to be better men and women—to be more successful, understanding, and diligent than they were before they became ill. These expectations, and the gratitude that was implicit in them, were often frustrated as patients regularly became angry, uncooperative, or depressed. The nurses' tendency was to retaliate as a result of anger and disappointment.

The nurses also developed strong feelings of possessiveness and overprotectiveness toward their patients. These feelings expressed themselves in resentment of new resident physicians, to whom the nurses had to make clear that "they are my patients," and in sabotaging the role of the unit psychiatrist because they felt someone was taking their patients away. Manifestations of overprotectiveness were also demonstrated in wishes to control patients' trips and struggles with family members over the performance of procedures.

Another of Kaplan De-Nour's group's findings that may relate to the overprotectiveness, and perhaps to overidentification as well, was the nurses' tendency to see dialysis patients as suffering much more than did the rest of the medical team on the unit. These feelings appear to be reflections of guilt experienced by the nurses and were often dealt with by attempts to "give" something to the patients. The nurses would often urge more frequent blood transfusions or give food and drink to patients although these were restricted.

INTERVENTION: HELPING THE PATIENT COPE WITH HEMODIALYSIS

Preventive Therapy

Patients starting on hemodialysis need to have practical goals set for their work, school, or household activity. It is important that the nurse enter into team decisions concerning goals of patients. As previously mentioned, the setting of unrealistic ones are among the stresses that many patients face. It is best to aim a bit low and to be delighted that the patient has attained a greater degree of rehabilitation than planned than to have the inverse occur.

Consideration also needs to be given to informing patients about the psychological complications of their illness and treatment. For example, since impotence seems to occur in at least 70% of all male patients, shouldn't all male patients be told of the possibility that this may occur? The author of this chapter generally thinks that it is best that patients be adequately prepared for possible complications, especially if the chance of their occurring seems reasonably certain or likely. Getting back to the example of impotence, the patient who has been told of the possibility of its occurring will tend to respond to its occurrence in a less anxiety-ridden way than the patient who is less well informed. The well-informed patient will tend to see his impotence as a complication of hemodialysis rather than as something in him that is innately defective and will more likely communicate his difficulties to professional staff, thus enabling earlier therapeutic intervention.

Early Diagnosis of Psychological Problems

It is important that all health professionals be adequately informed as to the psychological complications of hemodialysis. This information will enable health professionals to diagnose difficulties early in their course of treatment of patients so that therapy may be delivered sooner. Patients tend to hide their psychological problems, and informed professionals, by gentle inquiry, may encourage patients to share their problems with them. A head start is needed in knowing what some of these difficulties are, so that inquiries can be adequately directed.

Psychiatric Therapy

Although psychiatric problems are common among these patients, few patients tend to be in formal psychotherapy due, in part, to the fact that they, as a group, tend to be major deniers of their psychological problems. In addition, most hemodialysis patients feel "over-doctored." They are loath to get involved in any treatment modality that involves their spending additional time in a health care setting. Of course, there are many exceptions to this. In our experience, most psychotherapies need to take place actually within the hemodialysis setting, utilizing time spent on the machine for the therapy. Such a situation entails some compromise, since interruptions will occur and, at times, conversations may be overheard.

The use of psychiatric medications, the so-called psychotropics, may be helpful in many of these patients. As in the case of all medications, the contraindications are that nothing a dialysis patient receives should be primarily excreted by the kidney, lest it be accumulated in toxic levels, nor should it be dialyzable, lest it be removed and not attain therapeutic levels. Fortunately the tricyclic antidepressants and phenothiazines belong in neither of the interdicted groups. With depression as common as it is among these patients, it is our impression that the antidepressants should be much more widely used than they are.

Sexual Therapy

Concerning the sexual dysfunctions of these patients, there are newer forms of therapy that require the attention of all health professionals. Masters and Johnson behavioral techniques have potentially wide use among patients on hemodialysis. To understand this potential use, the concept of secondary sexual dysfunction needs to be understood. For example, if a 35-year-old juvenile-onset diabetic man experiences a single episode of impotence due to diabetic neuropathy, how it is perceived by him is crucial. If he sees this as a major blow to himself as a man, he may approach future sexual encounters with great doubts or withdraw entirely from them. If his masculine sense is well-based, he will have less psychological difficulty. Thus, a problem which is entirely organic in origin can have secondary psychological effects. This is also true of sexual dysfunctions that are purely psychological. They engender further doubts and further withdrawal. The methods of Masters and Johnson[22] and the modifications of Helen Singer Kaplan[23] essentially attempt to help patients re-enter the sexual sphere in a programmed, step-by-step manner. Recent studies show that these techniques can be most helpful among hemodialysis patients.[24,25] Their use by a wider group of health professionals is needed in order to deliver this treatment to a larger group of patients.

SUMMARY

Life on hemodialysis is an arduous one. It is one in which a patient is faced with the stresses common to all chronic illnesses, but with some peculiar to this life-saving medical treatment. The responses of patients to this treatment and its stresses vary greatly. There are many psychological problems of which the health care professional, especially the nurse, needs to be aware in order that the complications of hemodialysis may be discerned early and appropriate treatment delivered.

REFERENCES

1. Levy NB: Coping with Maintenance Hemodialysis-Psychological Considerations in the Care of Patients. *In* Massry SG, Sellers AL (eds): Clinical Aspects of Uremia and Dialysis. Springfield, Ill, Charles C. Thomas, pp. 53–68, 1976

2. Reichsman F, Levy NB: Problems in Adaptation to Maintenance Hemodialysis: A Four-Year Study of 25 Patients. Arch Int Med 128: 850–865, 1972

3. Eady RAJ: Why I Have Not a Kidney Transplant after Nine and One-Half Years as a Hemodialysis Patient. Transplant Proc 5: 1115–1117, 1973

4. Lefebre P, Norbert A, Crombez JC: Psychological and Psychopathological Reactions in Relation to Chronic Hemodialysis. Can Psych Assoc J 17: 9–11, 1972

5. Wright RG, Sand P, Livingston G: Psychological Stress During Hemodialysis for Chronic Renal Failure. Ann Intern Med 64: 611–621, 1966

6. Crammond WA, Knight PR, Lawrence JF: The Psychiatric Contribution to a Renal Unit Undertaking Chronic Haemodialysis and Renal Homo-transplantation. Br J Psych 113: 1201–1212, 1967

7. Foster FG, Cohn GL, McKegney FP: Psychobiologic Factors and Individual Survival on Chronic Renal Hemodialysis—A Two-Year Follow-Up: Part I. Psychosom Med 35: 64–82, 1973

8. Abram HS, Moore GI, Westervelt FB Jr: Suicidal Behavior in Chronic Dialysis Patients. Am J Psych 127: 1199–1204, 1971

9. Scribner BH: Panel. *In* Levy NB (ed): Living or Dying: Adaptation to Hemodialysis, Springfield, Ill, Charles C. Thomas, p. 5, 1974

10. McKegney FP, Lange P: The Decision to No Longer Live on Chronic Hemodialysis. Am J Psych 128: 267–274, 1971

11. Levy NB, Wynbrandt GD: The Quality of Life on Maintenance Hemodialysis. Lancet 1:1328–1330, 1975

12. Scribner BH: Panel. *In* Levy NB (ed): Living or Dying: Adaptation to Hemodialysis, Springfield, Ill, Charles C. Thomas, p. 25, 1974

13. Abram HS, Hester LR, Epstein GM, et al: Sexual Functioning in Patients with Chronic Renal Failure. J Nerv Ment Dis 160: 220–226, 1975

14. Levy NB: Sexual Adjustment to Maintenance Hemodialysis and Renal Transplantation: National Survey by Questionnaire. Trans Amer Soc Artif Int Organs 19:138–143, 1973

15. Massry SG, Goldstein DA, Procci WR, et al: Impotence in Patients with Uremia: A Possible Role for Parathyroid Hormone. Nephron 19: 305–310, 1977

16. Strauch M, Huber W, Rahauser G, et al: Rehabilitation in Patients Undergoing Maintenance Hemodialysis: Results of a Questionnaire in 15 Dialysis Centres. Trans EDTA 8: 28–33, 1971

17. Crammond WA, Knight PR, Lawrence JR: The Psychiatric Contribution to a Renal Unit Undertaking Chronic Hemodialysis and Renal Homo-transplantation. Br J Psych 113: 1201–1212, 1967

18. Levy NB: The Psychology and Care of the Maintenance Hemodialysis Patient. Heart and Lung 2: 400–405, 1973

19. Crammond WA, Knight PR, Lawrence JR, et al: Psychological Aspects Of Chronic Renal Failure. Br Med J 1: 539–543, 1968

20. Kaplan De-Nour A, Czaczkes JW: Emotional Problems and Reactions of the Medical Care Team in a Chronic Hemodialysis Unit. Lancet 2: 987–991, 1968

21. Kaplan De-Nour A, Czaczkes JW: Professional Team Opinion and Professional Bias—A Study of a Hemodialysis Team. J Chron Dis 24: 533–541, 1971

22. Masters W, Johnson V: Human Sexual Inadequacy, Boston, Little Brown, 1970

23. Kaplan HS: The New Sex Therapy, New York Quadrangle/The New York Times Book Company, 1974

24. Berkman AH: Sex Counseling with Hemodialysis Patients. Dial Transplant 7: 924–927, 1978

25 McKevitt PM: Role of the Nephrology Social Worker in Treating Sexual Dysfunction. Dial Transplant 7: 928–942, 1978

CHAPTER 13

The Respiratory Intensive Care Unit: Problems, Conflicts, and Potential Resolutions

Peter G. Tuteur

The respiratory intensive care unit is a complex social organization. Patterns of interaction initially are preset according to a functional stratification system, but over time this interaction mode is mediated by personal variables: response is to the person, not simply the status or position. At the center of the system is the patient. Other participants in the social system include nurses, physicians, the patient's family, and a wide variety of professional and nonprofessional support staff. The microcosmic society is a dynamic one; individuals enter and exist almost constantly. Their sojourn may be very brief (for just a few minutes), intermittent but regular (eight hours a day, five days a week, sometimes for years), or prolonged (twenty-four hours a day for days, weeks, or months). Nurses continually interact with each other, administrative staff, the patient, the patient's family, and the medical staff. Potential for conflict is great. For each general category of interaction is a table that lists potential problems and conflicts and their solutions.

The following narrative depicts activities centered around a fictional five-bed respiratory intensive care unit; the vignette illustrates some of the points outlined in tabular form. It is printed on the right half of each page. Marginal comments and references to the tables are located to the left. They are not intended to be all-inclusive, but to serve as a guide and to facilitate discussion.

The story begins: It is 6:00 a.m. on a mid-September morning. The fall-laden air has left behind the heat of summer, but the respiratory virus season has yet to begin. The Respiratory Intensive Care Unit of this teaching hospital has one empty bed. Newly assigned graduate nurses all have received congratulatory letters following their licensure exam; competition for these nursing positions in the RICU was stiff. The new interns finally seemed more effective after they had bolstered four years of medical school with a few months of practical experience. As the light from the rising sun filters through the partially closed blinds, the night nurses are making final preparations for report: morning blood gases drawn, I&Os finalized, vital signs entered on the chart.

Table V
Knowledgeable nurse associated with inexperienced physician

Mr. Jones in A bed requests to be bagged and is repeatedly hitting the tabletop bell on his night stand as if he were desk clerk calling for a sleeping bellhop. "I'll be right there, Mr. Jones," calls Terry, in a practiced and comforting stage whisper. Terry appreciates Fred Jones' paroxysms of dyspnea. Even though he is receiving oxygen sufficient to improve his blood gases to nearly normal, the severity of his interstitial fibrosis and the stiffness of his lungs yearn for hyperinflation and precipitate his panic reaction. The house staff is looking vigorously for a specific diagnosis, though Terry knows the odds of finding a treatable one are minuscule.

Table III
Demanding patient

Table V
Physician and nurse differ about optimal clinical plan

Fred Jones has been in the RICU for almost a week now. He was referred to the teaching hospital by his long-time family physician, an elderly man who practices in the farming community where Fred lives. Fred told Terry about the seemingly interminable ride in the ambulance past miles of cornfields during harvest to the strange city and its even less familiar hospital. More than the physical unknown, Fred feared the inevitable conclusions of the specialists. As he was ringing his bell, he suspected that Terry, even with a long weekend coming, probably would be the most empathic of the staff. But even empathy sometimes doesn't help.

Table I
Good leadership

It is now 6:26 a.m. Nearly a whole shift's work of charting has to be completed; report has to be dictated into the tape recorder (a good innovation of a strong head nurse, Margaret). Fred wants one last bit of hyper-inflation and some psychological support. Terry, too, needs psychological support. After an early May vacation, there was a great deal of overtime during June, July, and August while the new graduates were oriented and the more senior staff took their holidays. By now Terry felt "burned out" and the head nurse, Margaret, had suggested a long weekend. Terry was packed and ready for a woodland adventure in Brown County—no phones, no bells, no alarms, no other demands; just a few more tasks to complete. Fred could wait—but Terry couldn't wait to help Fred.

Table II
Uninterrupted
RICU routine

Suddenly Terry's thoughts were interrupted by the clanging of flesh on tubular aluminum. The "underdose" (as such patients were unaffectionately dubbed by JD, one of the more senior members of the nursing staff) was waking up, attempting to reject the taped nasotracheal tube while playing John Cage on the side rails, using swinging upper extremities covered with leather restraints. "SHIT!" muttered JD in a cultured Southern twang, "Ms. Pearlstein has to pick this time finally to clear her Doriden soup. Terry, come help me tie this spoiled brat down. She'll destroy every line and give us more work if we don't get her down."

Terry knew exactly how JD felt. Last night, when Leah Pearlstein was admitted, it was Terry who helped care for her.

Hours of work in an effort to help save someone who wanted to destroy herself always rekindled this unresolved conflict. Terry was trained to help the sick, but religious teachings condemned suicide, drugs, and alcohol. Almost reflexively Terry dropped everthing, forgetting about report and Fred, and helped JD securely restrain Ms. Pearlstein. Why did a young woman with an M.A. in archaeology and three years digging for relics in Israel come home only to behave in such a manner? A brief visit with her concerned, anxious, and affluent parents provided no insight. Terry made the best of the interruption by going over to Fred briefly, patting him on the back, and slowly hyperventilating him with the Ambu bag. It is interesting how it seemed like just a couple of unsatisfying breaths to him, yet a slow, tedious, unending process to Terry. Just then it was Margaret who looked into the 150-square-foot cubicle. "How are you doing, Terry?"

Table III
Repugnant patient

Table III
Direct patient care responsibilities juxtaposed to paper work

"O.K. I still have a lot to do before report."

"Gee, Fred, you look much better today. Let me bag you while Terry finishes up some of the remaining work. You know there's a long weekend coming up and we surely don't want to delay it."

Table I
Effects of strong leadership

Margaret, only four years Terry's senior, always seemed to know what to do to support her staff. It wasn't the big decisions that established Margaret's reputation as a strong head nurse. It was the day-to-day empathy, not only for patients but also for staff, her fairness, and her understanding that kept things moving at a highly positive level in this potential pressure cooker. Her action was the boost Terry needed to finish up, dictate report, and head out in search of clean autumn air.

As Margaret finished bagging Fred, she planned the sequence of her immediate activities. She would check the other three patients in the unit quickly. She needed only a few seconds to absorb everything in the room, determining that all alarms were in the "on" position and all IVs, nasogastric tubes, catheters, endotracheal tubes, ventilators, IVACS, and everything else functional. She took a quick look at the STAT book to be prepared with recent laboratory data when the onslaught of physicians hit—attending, pulmonary fellow, residents, interns, four-year students, third-year students. Also, she knew that she would have to talk to JD today: he was getting a little too cynical and some of his cynicism was rubbing off on the younger nurses. JD would be leaving soon, starting nurse anesthetic school. He might not have to interact with patients then, but, for now, Margaret wasn't going to let him undo what had taken her years to build up.

Table II
Hypercritical attitude associated with prolonged RICU assignment

Seated so quietly in the corner as almost to be overlooked was Courtney McCormick. Nurse McCormick had the easiest assignment of the night shift: her patient was Allison Cone, the patient in E bed. Mrs. Cone, the 62-year-old president of the League of Women Voters, had required mechanical ventilation for the past three months. Mrs. Cone usually slept well at night, especially since the physicians recently recognized what the nurses had known for several weeks: She was never going to get off the ventilator. Courtney was a good nurse, skillful, energetic, yet only empathic with those patients of a social class to which she herself aspired. The scuttlebut was that Courtney could sit for hours talking to Mrs. Cone while other nurses were inundated with the never-ending respon-

Table V
Physician and nurse differ about optimal clinical plan

Table III
Social status

sibilities of acutely ill patients. It was speculated that she even could do so while a patient in the next bed arrested.

Report is over. Fred is ready for breakfast. Ms. Pearlstein is waking up. Mrs. Cone is ready for another day, allowing her to mourn the loss of spontaneous ventilation and prepare herself for continuous mechanical ventilation at home. JD's other patient, Dr. Robert Baker, an anesthesia resident recovering from Guillain-Barré, is to be discharged from the unit today; a party is planned. C bed is unoccupied, the starched white linen ready to be violated by a new "hit," as the house staff tended to call a new admission. The RICU now is bright with sunlight; the blinds are open. The day shift is arriving.

Table I
Leader makes a difficult decision

As the night shift left, only JD stayed behind, having volunteered to work two consecutive shifts when Darleen Delacroix called in "sick." Only hesitatingly did Margaret accept his voluntary assignment and then as a mixed blessing. The ER had already called with a potential "hit"; but JD surely was "burning out," manifested by not only his cynicism, but also his plans for a career change—anesthesiology school. Nevertheless, she needed his help to care for the patients. JD continued his assignment of Ms. Pearlstein and Dr. Baker, while the other two nurses on the day shift were listening to the tape-recorded reel. Dr. Pamela Herrington, a respected postgraduate pulmonary fellow, telephoned, announcing the imminent arrival of a new patient for C bed. Pam described him as a 48-year-old with well-documented, moderately advanced pulmonary disease, who had had a crush injury of his chest while working the night shift at a local steel foundry. He was intubated despite his combativeness.

Margaret immediately knew what to do: change JD's assignment to the new patient since Dr. Baker was going to be transferred. She rapidly told the story to JD as the ward clerk notified Respiratory Therapy about the need for a ventilator. Margaret had had some experience with crush injuries while she was a nurse on the surgical floor. The contusions to a previously normal lung were bad enough, but trauma superimposed on a preexisting obstructive airways disease meant long-term care at best.

Table I
Delegate responsibilities to the strong nurse

JD was pleased both with the assignment of an acutely ill patient who probably wouldn't be talking back to him and the confidence Margaret displayed in his abilities to care for an obviously difficult patient. He responded to this feeling by helping the respiratory therapist set up the ventilator. JD anticipated an order for mechanical ventilation with a moderate rate and generous volumes to try to prevent the patient from initiating a breath and inward movement of the fractured ribs caused by a negative intrathoracic pressure. He knew IMV was not indicated. In the old days, orthopedic fixation of the chest was used, but now, with a contemporary ventilator, this was unnecessary.

Table I
Strong nurse accepts difficult tasks

Suddenly, an eclectic team of white coats entered, pushing a gurney carrying Oscar Schwartzwald, the new patient. Trailing not far behind was Dr. T. Barton Bright. As JD orchestrated the transfer of Mr. Schwartzwald from the gurney to C bed, Dr. Bright scurried around. Without even the slightest glance at the patient, he located the emergency room chart, ordered the ward clerk to secure the old records, and headed for the back conference room with pen in hand to read the chart. In contrast, Dr. Herrington exploited this patient care situation to do a little teaching. Instead of barking the ventilator orders, she asked for suggestions among not only house staff and students, but also the nursing personnel. As a junior student fumbled with the question about ventilator setting, Pamela gave JD a nod of approval when he flipped open the cover of the MA1, revealing his handiwork. As she attached the ventilator to the patient's size 8 endotracheal tube, she concisely and precisely explained the rationale for these settings. The departure of the ER personnel signaled an opportunity for a thorough physical exam. Pamela identified a previously undetected scalp laceration, pointed out the obviously flail chest, and explained the reason for her search for other soft tissue injury. She intended to speak with coworkers and family after she sought out the assigned intern, but he suddenly appeared in the small cubicle with interns' manual in hand asking JD,

Table V Excellent physician-health care team communication

"Are you the nurse here?"

Before JD could respond to Dr. Bright's introduction, more questions followed. "Who set up this ventilator without my permission? Who the hell do you think is in charge here? Don't you know a hundred percent oxygen is a toxin? What are you trying to do, poison the patient? Wait until the Chief Resident hears about this!"

Table V Inappropriate M.D.

Halfway through her heel-oriented pirouette, Pamela calmly, though forcefully, broke the hushed silence created by the gasps of the assembled colleagues by saying "I'm Pamela Herrington, the pulmonary fellow. I assume you're the intern on Team 4."

"That's right," T.B. retorted.

"How about sitting down and discussing the problems here so that we can have a unified approach to help this patient."

It took Pamela only a few minutes to establish credibility and soothe this highly intelligent and highly insecure young man. A plan was established and executed with effectiveness. About an hour later, things were stable and JD took a coffee break.

He looked at Margaret and, beyond ear shot of anybody else, commented "You should have seen her take care of that little shit; he was ready to pull a power play and, before he knew it, he had ten minutes of penalty time, had his stick taken away, and he was down on his hands and knees begging for help. She's one hell of a doctor. Let me tell you all these interns are classic examples of the Peter Principle."

Margaret knew that she couldn't let this conversation continue. JD was physically tired and venting. Soon it would degenerate into a cynical tirade against Intensive Care Units, self-abuse, hospital administration, and a strong central government.

Table I
Differing opinions and strong leadership

Margaret said, "You know, JD, you surely are entitled to your viewpoints. And I agree that Dr. Herrington is a competent consultant and that Dr. Bright is a little immature, but it's counterproductive to blow this totally out of perspective. Our job here is to provide the best care for the patients. Granted, this is only your temporary goal now in the RICU, but you are staying in medicine and hopefully you will have your niche in anesthesiology. In the last three or four weeks that you are here I think it would be best for you, us, and our patients just to keep it cool—a little more restraint with respect to expressing your thoughts. I know you understand; you have been around a long time."

JD had to have the last word, "Shit, Margaret! I'll miss you!"

The crises were over, but Margaret still needed to check Marilyn Marrow, who was assigned to Leah Pearlstein. Marilyn came with high grades and recommendations detailing what a good student she was. Margaret felt she couldn't go against the excellent paper critieria, yet, on interview, there was something missing. Maybe she was immature, in contrast to her stylish apparel, which seemed directly out of *Vogue*.

Leah Pearlstein's doctors extubated her during the arrival of the new patient. As Margaret approached the cubicle housing D bed, Ms. Pearlstein, and her nurse, the conversation sounded more appropriate to Elizabeth Arden's fashionable beauty boutique than to an RICU.

"Yes, Ms. Pearlstein, we will get you presentable before Dr. Hunter visits. Of course, we will call his office to remind them that you will not be able to make your usual 2:00 appointment. Yes, I called the hostess of the luncheon at the Museum; she wished you a speedy recovery! Which robe would you prefer to wear this morning?"

Yet this bizzare conversation didn't prepare Margaret for what she saw! Margaret was shocked when she entered. There was Marilyn Marrow, R.N., kneeling on the floor next to the armchair in which Ms. Pearlstein reigned in the Pucci robe, and she was manicuring her patient's nails. JD, walking by en route to the cabinet for supplies, did an honest double take. If it hadn't been for his earlier conversation with Margaret and the entrance of the elder Pearlsteins, an uncensored JD comment might have been forthcoming. But Margaret broke the tension with "Miss Marrow, why don't you let Leah visit with her parents?" In the solitude of the back room Margaret continued. "Marilyn, what were you doing? Was that health care?"

"I was just trying to make her comfortable. She was worried about how she would look when the psychiatrist comes. What's his name, Dr. Hunter?"

Table III
Inappropriate behavior in a clinical setting

"Marilyn, your motivation is good, but do you perceive your patient's problem as how to get her social schedule in line with her activities as a patient in the RICU?"

"Well, no, but . . . . "

"Often, it's difficult to put things into perspective, but it shouldn't be too difficult to understand that your patient, Leah, purposefully swallowed a lethal dose of Doriden 36 hours ago! She wanted to kill herself."

"I just wanted to help. She's such a wonderful person, and young!"

"Marilyn, you're a nurse now. Yes, it's important to make your patients more comfortable, but comfort, too, has professional implications. You can do more than a manicurist or candy striper. Remember, the problem is that Leah felt so negative about herself that she attempted self-destruction. The question to you, then, is why? Has the acute episode been controlled? What about the future? Prevention, therapy, continuing care?"

"I understand, I think . . . . but, what should I do now? Do I tell her that I shouldn't do her nails and that I'm to interview her with respect to the circumstances about her attempted suicide?"

"Oh! Come on! No! Finish her nails, but as you do so, in an open-ended, almost

Table III
Constructive criticism

informal way, begin to find out about her and the circumstances surrounding her suicide attempt. Did she know what she was doing? Try it, that's the correct approach." As they walked back to the bedside together, Margaret patted Marilyn on the shoulder; Mr. Pearlstein, greeted Margaret with the authority of one who usually commands the respect of others.

"Ms."

"Yes, sir!" responded Margaret automatically.

"Would you please make sure that Ms. Pearlstein get transferred to a suite in Ford Tower Pavillion, preferably one with an Eastern exposure?"

Table IV
Need for education of family about patient's problem

"Mr. Pearlstein, please come into my office," she said aloud, while thinking, "I've got to get him on my turf." Margaret began to explain the elements of the clinical situation and asked Leah's father about the whys? ever befores? etc. Dr. Herrington joined the dialogue a few minutes later, adding credibility to the discussion. As Mr. Pearlstein left, he was a shade paler. He apparently realized the severity of his daughter's actions for the first time. Leah was not to be a sojourner in the health care scene, but a permanent resident. Leah's past psychiatric treatment had been viewed by the family as a "phase," almost a socially predictable event. This suicide attempt, or "gesture" as a friend had called it, reflected a more fundamental and serious pathology. Marilyn's actions, too, reflected an attitude similar to Mr. Pearlstein's. Interestingly, both now viewed the patient in a more realistic way.

It was Margaret's turn for a break. Usually she retreated to the back conference room and brewed a cup of tea, made by filling a metallic perforated "egg" with her own special blend of semiexotic teas. This was a luxury that she now accorded herself. Such a stay in the back conference room allowed other personnel to come in and air problems. As suddenly as the small teapot began to whistle and shake on the portable hotplate in the corner of the room, it abruptly halted, as Rachel Regan lifted it off its berth to fill Margaret's cup.

Rachel, who was in her second RICU year, had done quite well. She rapidly learned the specialized manual skills necessary to be an effective intensive care nurse. This, superimposed on several years of general nursing experience and an unusual sense of maturity and sensitivity, allowed Margaret to peg her as someone with a great deal of growth potential.

"Margaret, I've been thinking. I really like Mrs. Cone. She's a dear little old lady. But, what are we actually doing for her? She's very aware now that she has no potential to resume the life she desires to live. At best, she can look forward to staying in her room at home attached to a ventilator, never again participating actively in her political affairs. On the other hand, someone said her hospital bill was almost $120,000. If she goes home, it might be cut down to $10,000 or $15,000 a month with round-the-clock nurses and rental of all that equipment. Margaret, what are we doing?"

Table III
Perceived poor cost-effectiveness of health care plan

"We're taking care of people. The attention and the care we have given Mrs. Cone gives her a feeling that people care. Her family has been attentive. She can take pride in the success of her husband and daughters. She can relish the future of her grandchildren. She can read and contribute to her friends and even her organization. I don't think that we, as nurses or as members of the health care profession, can attempt to set a dollar value on this outcome. Is it cost-effective to society? I don't know. Is it cost-effective for Mrs. Cone? It must be, for she has planned her health care by buying the best insurance available. She has paid for this up front and is now cashing in."

"You're talking as if health care is an unlimited resource."

"In our hospital and in our unit, essentially it is. I'm not a health care economist or planner. I'm a nurse, and I view my responsibilities as caring for individual patients in the best way I know how."

By this time, Margaret's tea had cooled and she faced the conflict of making another cup laced with the guilt of a prolonged break. "Hell," Margaret thought, "this was a professional discussion and now I can take a real break."

There was momentary calm in the back room. Margaret sat alone. Two noises broke the silence: one was the shrieking whistle of the teakettle; the other was the unmistakable alarm of the cardiac monitor. It was no false alarm. Mr. Schwartzwald had arrested! Margaret pushed the teakettle off the hotplate and the whistling sound diminished, both because of the cooling effect and the widening distance between the kettle and Margaret's ears, as she virtually flew to C bed. Marilyn was ushering Mrs. Schwartzwald into a waiting area. JD had initiated all the appropriate resuscitative efforts. Dr. Herrington seemed to have come out of nowhere, assessing the situation and initiating the "code." Then, as Dr. Bright continued to conduct the code, he clearly appreciated the supervision of Pamela Herrington. Dramatically, the flat ECG transformed to normal electrical activity and the patient was saved, for the moment.

Again Pamela exploited the situation for education. She initiated a discussion with Dr. Bright, the assembled physicians, and students about the medical and social implications of the recent events. In an open, yet controlled, discussion she developed the concepts that to interact effectively with the family, one must use a great deal of empathy and sensitivity. Stressed was the fact that the recent events occurred quite suddenly, leaving too little time for the development of defense mechanisms or even the initiation of a mourning process. A candid approach with a great deal of support was decided upon and Dr. Bright became the self-appointed liaison between the health care group and the family. Bolstered by the discussion, he handled it admirably.

Today, the shift will end in an unusual way. The customary influx of four or five nurses wearing crisp white uniforms will be augmented by many others and their friends to help Dr. Baker celebrate his discharge from the unit. He is to be transferred to a general floor, following a prolonged stay in the RICU recovering from Guillain-Barré. Attendance was usually very good at these parties, for it was a time not only to join the patient in the ceremonial departure, but also to express, in a socially acceptable way, self-satisfaction. Cookies, Hawaiian punch, salty peanuts, and a variety of ethnic dishes reflecting the origins of the team graced an old wooden table rejuvenated by a clean white tablecloth marred only by an India ink imprint of the name and logo of the teaching hospital. Following a brief peak of excitement, people filtered out, leaving the evening shift to clean up and begin the

Table III
Celebration of success

care of the four remaining patients. They awaited a "hit" to B bed, empty for the first time in many weeks.

Epilogue

It is now a couple of years later. The physical facilities of the RICU belie any passage of time. Many of the characters, however, are changed. It is 0630 and the nursing staff is winding down after a rather uneventful night. With a needlepoint-decorated briefcase in hand, Terry briskly walked into the unit. She warmly greeted the staff, stabled her belongings, and talked with each patient as she walked from cubicle to cubicle. A glance at the STAT book confirmed what she already knew—no major disasters had occurred during the night. As the change of shift approached, eight or ten nurses congregated in the conference room.

"Terry! We've got a problem with the front office again," one complained.

"Tell me about it."

"Remember, we arranged the schedule so that I could work three weekends in a row and convert the last weekend off to a four-day vacation. Well, the schedule came up from downstairs and they assigned me to cover a general medical floor for someone else. Terry, you know how important this is to me . . . "

"Don't worry. Continue to plan for that weekend. I'll take care of it."

Terry knew that her former head nurse would be empathic. She only hoped, at this late date, that something could be done about the schedule.

It almost seemed like a blessing that everything else went so smoothly this morning. In part, Terry assumed, it was due to the fact that winter was over and that spirits, as well as skill level, were up. After some self-debate, she decided on a chance meeting with Margaret during a cafeteria lunch.

Almost like a Hollywood movie script, Margaret and Terry met at the cafeteria's entrance. No formal arrangement had been made; no appointment was necessary. As they walked through the line, they exchanged small talk about Terry's winter trip to the Bahamas and Margaret's new child. It was Margaret who selected a table in the far corner away from the main stream of lunchtime traffic. "You know, Terry, one thing I learned in the past six months, working down in the administrative offices of the nursing department, is that many people forget what it is like up there taking care of patients."

"Really?"

"For example, someone, and no one is willing to admit it, changed Mabel Hodges' schedule, converting her long weekend at the end of the month into an assignment on the general ward. Did you know that?"

"Yes, Margaret; you forget I had training under an excellent nurse."

Table II Good administrative response

"Well, Terry, you can just tell Mabel that the revised schedule will be out by the end of the day and she has nothing to worry about."

"I already did!"

Both women smiled. Terry realized what an asset it was to have Margaret in the nursing office. She could picture how difficult it might have been dealing with a totally unsympathetic paper pusher. On the other hand, she felt a little sorry for Margaret, who had accepted the position only reluctantly so that her hours might best coincide with her family obligations. Just then, Margaret's beeper went off. It relayed a message that the Patient Care Committee Meeting was canceled.

"Terry, the Patient Care Committee Meeting can be canceled but as long as we have people like you taking care of patients, at least patient care will continue as scheduled."

This scenario is designed to heighten awareness of the many problems and conflicts that may occur in an RICU, where people with a variety of individual conflicts and defense mechanisms interact as they focus on a single important subject—the patient. It is only with such awareness and sensitivity that problems can be minimized and conflicts resolved so that energies can be directed where they belong—to promote optimal and intensive health care to very sick patients.

TABLE I. Nurse-Nurse Interaction

Situation	*Potential Problem*	*Approaches to Solution*
Each patient is assigned a different nurse each shift	Lack of unified nursing approach	Assign compatible nurses to a specific patient. Schedule open discussion about "the patient." Encourage precise physician orders. Make clear and available policy statements.
Differing opinions among staff concerning solutions to specific, recurrent, clinical problems	Hostile disagreement about solutions to patient problems	Schedule presentation of data in seminar format. Get respected authority to help resolve problems. Anticipate the problem and have leader discuss it before the fact. Have good leadership.
Strong vs. weak nurse	Weaker nurse is dominated and becomes "scapegoat"; her morale and performance drop	Schedule private and individual conferences to discuss performance and skills with head nurse. Develop a plan for skill improvement, using assignments requiring skills initially simple but progressing to the more complex. Place weaker nurse in potential success situations to build up confidence.
	Strong nurse NOT delegated more complex responsibilities, yielding substandard performance	Leader must be aware of situation and should assign strong nurse to appropriate responsibilities.
Lack of leadership	Existence of a variety of opinions regarding policy without any consensus. Leadership developing in a nonleadership position, adding to conflict	Only solution: get effective leader in a leadership position (head nurse, medical director); delegate responsibility to head nurse for personnel change.

TABLE II. Nurse-RICU (Administration)

Situation	*Potential Problem*	*Approaches to Solution*
Large staff and undesirable working hours	Perception that an individual's work schedule is more undesirable than that of colleagues	Leaders should convey a sense of fairness with assignments. Have long-range work plan. Have nurse-nurse support with respect to exchanging assignments.
	"Burn out"—indifference —overwork	Anticipate and schedule long weekends or vacation; refuse overtime.
Excessive strength required for tasks; long hours	Physical fatigue	Assign nurse to patients whose requirements are physically less demanding. Make more effective use of orderlies.
Isolation of administrative staff	Perception of lack of "nursing office" support	Foster effective communication by the administrative group of any decisions affecting RICU and by attendance by administrative personnel at general meetings.
Prolonged daily assignment to an intensive care unit without significant interruption	"ICUitis"—loss of fondness for RICU as professional niche; hypercritical attitude; search for job relocation	Arrange for physical departure from ICU for over 2 months within every 24 months; can be done either with continuing education, personal leave, or brief transfer to another nursing situation.
Realization that ideal and practical do not always coincide in daily activity	Frustration	Develop insight through individual conferences and group seminars, as well as informal discussion.

TABLE III. Nurse-Patient

Situation	*Potential Problem*	*Approaches to Solution*
"Uncooperative" patient	Refusal of treatment considered by health care team to be required for patient; i.e., refuses p.o. fluids, unrealistically limits exercise, reluctantly accepts or even refuses scheduled diagnostic or therapeutic activities	Have team discussion and support of primary nurse; additional support voiced to patient by a leader (M.D., head nurse); if unsuccessful, work around patient-imposed restrictions.
"Demanding" patient	Patient requests more nursing service than what is perceived as medically required	Have discussion between nurse and patient to allow patient to correctly anticipate response to "demands."
Nurse required to perform activity which is perceived, in an objective medical sense, to be appropriate but associated with negative emotional feelings or other duties	Need to perform necessary physiotherapy and postural drainage, which increases patient discomfort and nurse anxiety	Help nurse deal with anxiety. Closely monitor objective signs.
	Selection to complete medically less important duties before direct patient care responsibilities	Develop ability to establish priorities.

TABLE III. Nurse-Patient (Continued)

Situation	*Potential Problem*	*Approaches to Solution*
Socially repugnant patient—alcohol, tobacco, food, drug abuse	Conflict between desire to help person and to punish him as an offender of nurse's personal standards	Develop nurse's awareness of conflict; stress professional responsibility and measurement of clinical outcome.
Patient and nurse of different race, religion, sex	Range from indifference to discomfort to antagonism in caring for patient	Develop nurse's awareness of conflict. Balance patient assignment—during in-service training, stress the need to develop and maintain a professional attitude with all patients.
Social status apposition: patient and nurse	Extreme positive or negative attitude	Develop nurse's awareness of actions associated with conflict.
Perceived poor cost-effectiveness of health care plan	Perception of taking nurse time away from patient where efforts are perceived as more cost-effective	Discuss and stress responsibility to care for patient according to contemporary standards.
Inappropriate clinical behavior; nursing error	Self-depreciation vs. denial	Make objective assessment of care in retrospect; learn from mistakes; goal: avoid "mistake" in future. Express general concern to family. Also have open discussion with head nurse/medical director and general discussion (without incrimination) with staff; treat as stimulus for learning and self-improvement.
Success	Inability to display success; self-depreciation	Provide situation where success can be displayed in socially acceptable way.

TABLE IV. Nurse-Family

Situation	*Potential Problem*	*Approaches to Solution*
Enforcement of visiting regulation	Desire of family to see patient vs. nurses' time requirement to render care	Establish visiting guidelines, not strict regulations, and reinforce that "we all want best for patient"—counsel nurse to "see other side."
Family unaware of "rules" of unit	Family's "disobeying" rules is viewed by nurses as not appreciating health care efforts of staff	Give written information re RICU to family; personal orientation to family—reinforce as necessary; display empathy.
Discharge	Family confused—perceived rejection by RICU; developed dependency on RICU	Arrange for patient and family education—both general and disease-specific. Have formal set-up for RICU staff to continue to visit patients in new hospital location.
Death	Family places blame for fatality on doctors, nurses, and health care team	Support family's appropriateness of actions toward patient. Do not become defensive with family. Continue to show empathy.
Need for education of family about patient's problem	Inappropriate and potentially deleterious behavior by family	Arrange for honest appraisal of clinical situation with family by members of health care team.

TABLE V. Nurse-Doctor

Situation	*Potential Problem*	*Approaches to Solution*
Specialized nurse knowing more than M.D.—house staff	Inappropriately defensive doctor ordering nurse to perform what is perceived to be an inappropriate health care activity	Validate point of conflict with superior. Give objective data in professional manner. In extreme situation, inform M.D. that orders will not be carried out. Solicit help of medical director.
Uncooperative and/or inappropriately noncommunicative M.D.	Unclear directions or orders—"oral orders"	First, attempt direct communication with "uncooperative" doctor. Solicit help of head nurse, medical director, or other supervisor.
Clinical picture viewed differently by physician and nurse. Often this is due to the different amount of time each spends with patient	Discrepancy re therapeutic plan—often with respect to goal, activity, potential for weaning, patient cooperation	Develop rapport with physician and establish credibility of nurse observation. Have physician "educated" re potential problem.

CHAPTER 14

A Family Affair: Dealing with Families of ICU Patients

Nathan M. Simon and Gail Poelker

The emergence of *Intensive Care Units* (ICUs) as the setting for the application of highly specialized treatment programs for the critically ill has been a stimulus for the development of new and sophisticated treatment techniques and technologies. The new techniques and technologies have not only been in electronic equipment, specialized medical hard- and software, new medications, and medication schedules, but they also have included new nursing strategies. Programs to deal with the special needs of families of the ICU patient are examples of this latter type of development.

The impetus for the development of programs for the families of ICU patients derives from several sources.

1. The recognition that family members constitute an important part of the patient's environment during the ICU stay and that the interaction among patient, family member, and nurse can be either a positive or negative factor in this environment.
2. A need to quickly orient family members to the special ICU environment and its rules and regulations.
3. A response to human needs of the family members.
4. The broad interface of action that occurs between family members and ICU nursing personnel may have a considerable impact on the nurse's performance.
5. A recognition that misinformation and myths can develop quickly from exchanges among families during the time they are together in the waiting room.

6. A recognition that educational and rehabilitative efforts reduce disability after discharge and need to begin in the hospital and include family members.

The crises that result from patient entry into an ICU most often bring more family members to the hospital for longer periods of time. The ICU differs from most nursing units in hospitals in that access to the patient is subjected to more regulation—regulation that, in almost all cases, is nurses' responsibility to supervise. Where visiting rules are rigid and narrowly defined, it is the nurse who becomes the enforcer. Where rules allow for more exceptions and interpretations, it is most often the nurse who will make the decision about such interpretations.

REVIEW OF THE LITERATURE

The literature describing ICU experiences is notably deficient in references to family members' behavior and how it impacts on the patient and nurse. Michaels'[1] article on the psychological stress on the ICU nurse is one of the few that addresses the subject directly. Her report is an impressionistic study based, in large part, on her own experiences as an ICU nurse and on a survey of an undefined sample of ICU nurses and their attitudes towards patients and families. Michaels' starting point is the high state of stress under which ICU nurses function most often, and the frequency with which this can lead to feelings of depletion, depression, and exhaustion that can make the nurse unable to provide support to either patient or family member. She perceptively points out the ambivalence that frequently characterizes nurses' feelings to the families of ICU patients. Her study revealed that, while nurses say that they recognize family members as important and that they wish to help them, they also frequently believe family members should be kept out of the ICU. Some believe that ICU waiting rooms should be located far from the ICU, and families should stay away completely because being near causes the families "much anxiety." Michaels believes that, while nurses say they see their roles as supporters and comforters of the families, they also "invent" reasons to avoid interaction with families. Michaels offers little in the way of remedies for the problem she so accurately identifies. "Support" for the nurses is a concept that she does not define. She does suggest that "planned withdrawal" from especially stressful patients is possible as a way to enhance nurses' coping ability.

West[2] describes ICU stresses that affect patients, family, and staff. He identifies the ambivalence experienced by families who, on the one hand, are stressed because their family member has a life-threatening illness and, at the same time, are grateful because their relative is receiving the best care available. West also comments on the stress that visiting limitations places on families who most often wish to be close to the relative during his or her critical illness. West goes on to point out that family members are acutely aware that they will get more information from ICU personnel if they are actually in the patient's room and that they are often more comfortable seeing the situation first-hand rather than having it reported to them by nursing personnel. However, family members are also stressed by the ICU environment and the agony of their relatives and other patients. West offers a number of suggestions that involve architectural and design issues, group meetings for nursing personnel, and increased visiting privileges.

Ryan[3] describes a setting in which a program has been developed to deal with one specific aspect of relations with family members. She describes a hospital in which a psychiatric nurse is a part of the cardiac arrest team. The nurse's assignment is to stay with the family during the crisis. Ryan describes the goals of the nurse in this situation as: (1) to prevent distortion of the reality of the situation by the family; (2) to identify support persons for the family; and (3) to enhance family coping mechanisms.

Cooper[4], an ER nurse, writes an agonized, moving, autobiographical account of the ICU waiting room experience. In ten paragraphs she evokes the pain, helplessness, boredom, loneliness, and hatred that are generated in the ICU waiting room. One point that emerges from her paper is the hatred and jealousy that can be directed to nursing personnel because the nurses have ready access to the patient while the family member is often barred by the sign on the door that regulates visiting. The feelings she evokes most clearly are the pain, frustration, and anger of enforced passivity, and the loneliness and jealousy engendered by lack of contact.

Skelton and Dominian[5] studied 65 wives of men admitted to a CCU. Feelings of loss, guilt, and depression were common at the time of infarction. Wives formed attitudes toward the illness that influenced the way they reacted and treated their husbands at home. The wife's inability to communicate freely with her husband makes it useful to have reliable alternative sources to whom feelings can be expressed.

PATIENT-FAMILY-NURSE INTERACTION IN THE ICU

The reasons for developing specific programs for family members of ICU patients were identified in the introductory paragraphs of this paper. Following are a number of typical examples of problems in patient-family-nurse relations seen on a Medical Intensive Care Unit (MICU).

Family Overprotectiveness

One of the most frequent situations that makes an ICU nurse aware of the clinical implications of the family contact evolves out of the family's overprotectiveness. Families often see their patient as too sick to ambulate, wash, feed, or shave himself. They communicate this to the patient in both overt and subtle ways and to the nursing staff in styles that can be plaintive, hostile, or accusatory. When not dealt with appropriately, this can lead to increased anxiety and tension among patient/family/and nurse.

A 60-year-old single white male was admitted to the MICU with a diagnosis of myocardial infarction (MI). The patient had been a resident of a home for the aged for 10 years, primarily because of mild retardation. The patient's 84-year-old mother became a "full-time" waiting room occupant. She never missed a regular visiting period. If she visited at mealtime, she would insist on trying to feed the patient. The patient would be quite willing to let his mother do this and a clear pattern of increasing dependency was developing. The nurse caring for the patient took time to talk with the mother alone and explain the importance of letting the patient feed himself. This had an immediate positive short-term effect.

But the next day the patient's mother became upset and complained anxiously in the presence of the patient if the patient got out of bed to go to the toilet or to walk in his room. The mother insisted that the patient should be carried or moved in a wheel-chair. Her agitation visibly upset the patient and made him unsure about the increase in physical activity. Again, the nurse conferred alone with the mother and tried to deal with the patient's physical anxiety. Again, this had a short-term beneficial effect. But it became clear that each nursing intervention with the mother had only a transitory effect and that a long-established pattern of overprotectiveness, colored by a marked shared anxiety, was going to continue. Reports from the regular nursing division, to which the patient was eventually transferred, confirmed this.

Another frequent area of conflict is around family response to patients' eating patterns.

A 75-year-old male had his first admission to the MICU with a diagnosis of myocardial infarction. Both his 70-year-old wife and a 35-year-old married daughter would hover over the patient at mealtime and repeat over and over again that it was necessary for the patient to eat in order to get well. The mother and daughter continued to feed the patient even when he indicated disinterest in eating. They both appeared to be unaware of the patient's lack of appetite and moderate depression. His failure to clean his plate increased their anxiety and their efforts to get him to eat. Eventually the nurse made an attempt to deal with the situation when the wife and daughter were present. The daughter became upset at the nurse's straightforward explanation about illness and appetite. In the hall later, the daughter challenged the nurse and repeated her concern that her father was not eating enough. The nurse empathized with the daughter about her father's condition, reassured her about his lack of appetite, and re-explained reasons for not attempting to forcefeed the patient. With the repeated quiet, nonthreatening explanations, her anxiety decreased, as well as her challenging attitude to the nurse. The daughter's increase in understanding had a positive effect on the mother, who also became less anxious. Both refrained from making an issue of food for the remainder of the patient's stay on the MICU.

Family Concerns about Quality of Care

The issue of the quality of care is another frequent source of nurse/family interaction that affects all three units in the patient/family/nurse triad. Family anxiety that is not modulated is often expressed in criticisms about quality of care, such as accusations that nurses are not spending enough time with the patient or are not responding quickly enough to the patient's call lights. Sometimes criticisms of nursing care develop when families are not made clearly aware of the therapeutic program. Sedation of the highly anxious or disoriented patient or the need for restraints when chemical control of agitation is temporarily not feasible often are upsetting to families and can produce criticisms of the nursing staff.

A 60-year-old white male was admitted to the MICU from the SICU for treatment of mild respiratory failure. At admission, he was mildly disoriented, agitated, and verbally abusive. He made frequent attempts to climb out of bed. The patient's 50-year-old wife and 25-year-old son were extremely upset about the deterioration in the patient's condition that made the transfer necessary. Shortly after admission to the unit, the family began to make frequent trips to the nursing station to insist that a nurse stay in the room at all times. The nursing staff were providing adequate nursing care and were in the patient's room frequently. The patient's agitation and anxiety, in part exacerbated by the transfer, appeared to be moderating and controllable. However, the family's anxiety increased precipitously. They became increasingly hostile and critical of the nursing staff. They accused the nurses of not taking care of the patient. Despite numerous efforts to reassure the family and a great deal of time spent by the nurses with the family in an effort to respond to their anxiety, they persisted in their criticism and finally made arrangements for private duty nurses.

Patient-Family Interactions That Increase Patient Anxiety

Pathological and stressful interaction of family members and patients is regularly observed.

A 52-year-old male was admitted to the MICU with an arrhythmia (ventricular tachycardia). The nurse's initial contact with the wife and patient together, shortly after admission, led her to extend the regular visiting period. This arrangement made the patient extremely irritable. He began shouting at his wife to leave, angrily telling her she was breaking the hospital rules. He seemed frightened that "violation" of the hospital regulations would antagonize the staff and jeopardize his care. The nurse, still responding to her original empathic assessment of the marital interaction as a positive one, talked to the patient about the flexibility of the visiting rules. She assured him that it was all right with her and the rest of the nursing staff if the wife stayed for longer periods than the regular 15 minutes and she emphasized that the patient's wishes and needs were most important. The patient became calmer as the nurse talked and, when she finished, said in a subdued voice that he really wanted his wife to stay with him. The wife, who had become visibly upset and shaken by her husband's outburst, relaxed appreciably. During the remainder of the patient's MICU stay, the wife's visits were helpful in managing rather high levels of anxiety in the emotionally labile patient.

A 53-year-old woman, who had been widowed 6 years previously, was admitted to the MICU with severe pain. Admission diagnoses were: (1) Rule out MI; and (2) Hypertension. An MI was diagnosed shortly after admission. Mrs. L. was a nurse, but had not worked for several years. She consistently and steadfastly refused to acknowledge to any of the MICU nurses that she was a nurse and would become stubbornly silent if any nurse raised the subject. When attempts were made to do post-MI teaching, the patient denied knowing anything about medicines. She was hyperactive and resisted or behaved negatively to suggestions from the nursing staff, especially about rest and about restraining physical activity. She frequently was openly hostile and verbally abusive to the nursing staff, though more compliant with unit physicians.

The patient had three daughters, aged 16, 18, and 21. The daughters came only at regular visiting times and stayed for the allotted 15 minutes. As soon as the daughters entered her room, the patient and daughters would begin crying. The crying would be punctuated by angry accusations and counteraccusations by all parties involved in the visit. These visits retained their tumultuous character during her entire MICU stay.

One of the unit nurses finally came to understand that the patient was terrified of dying (one reason she persisted in being "ignorant" about things she had learned in her nursing career) and was concerned that her two younger daughters would have no one to support them. The patient was oscillating between massive denial and maladaptive hyperactivity as her primary ways of coping with the stress of her illness and the helplessness it imposed on her. The unit nurses began to respond to her differently. They tried to find ways for her to be realistically in control of her environment. They responded promptly and without argument when she ordered them to rearrange furniture in her room, adjust the blinds and lights, and reposition her bed. When she was transferred to a regular nursing division, her behavior changed dramatically. She had much more physical freedom and fewer restraints. She was pleasant and cooperative with the floor nurses and was friendly with the MICU nurses when she met them in the halls.

Positive Patient-Family Interactions

Many times nurses become aware of the positive effect of family/patient interaction.

A 63-year-old married man was hospitalized for myocardial infarction. His wife was 62. They had no children. It was his first infarction. Shortly after admission, the patient became agitated and then became disoriented, paranoid, and began to have ill-defined auditory hallucinations. He called for his wife frequently. The nurses observed that, while his wife was with the patient, he appeared better oriented and less anxious and made no mention of hallucinations. Psychiatric consultation with the patient revealed that he was oriented to time, place, and person. There were auditory hallucinations. He was markedly anxious. There was no evidence of organic brain syndrome. History revealed that the patient was very dependent on his wife. They had never been apart during forty years of marriage except for the time that he was at work. His wife made all the major decisions in their marriage. At the time this patient was hospitalized, the ICU visiting times were regulated very strictly to ten minutes out of every hour from 2 p.m. to 8 p.m. The recommendation was made to have the wife stay with the patient for longer periods of time. This would have been possible since the patient was in a private room, his condition was stable, and there were no special nursing problems. However, the director of the ICU refused to follow the recommendation, feeling that it would upset the family members of other patients who would not have as much visiting time with their patients on the ICU. Therefore, the patient was transferred off the ICU to a private room on a regular medical floor, where his symptoms disappeared completely and where he had an uneventful recovery.

A 55-year-old married male was admitted following a severe episode of gastrointestinal bleeding. The patient had developed severe respiratory distress growing out of marked muscle flaccidity following a cerebral vascular accident. The nurses quickly observed that the relationship that the patient had with his 52-year-old wife was a strong and positive one. The patient enjoyed having his wife with him and she was affectionate, stable, and direct with the patient in the time they spent together. The patient's wife was anxious during her visits, especially at times when she wanted to do something for her husband and felt unable to do so. Early in the patient's stay, the nursing staff began to involve the wife in the routine nursing care. They instructed her in back rubs, in proper techniques for turning, and in helping the patient with toileting. They also taught her to become aware of the signs that indicated a need for suctioning. The wife's participation in her husband's care was accompanied by a prompt decrease in anxiety. The wife and the nursing staff maintained an excellent working relationship over the three months the patient was on the unit. She became quite close to some of the nurses in a way that allowed her to openly share her personal burdens and at the same time permitted an intimacy growing out of mutual affection.

Family Distress and Poor Information Exchange

The lack of clear, concise, understandable information about the patient's condition, the treatment plan, and the equipment being used is another source of problems involving nurse/patient and family.

A 58-year-old white male was admitted to the MICU for the second time within a year with substernal pain three days after a cholecystectomy. The patient's condition fluctuated during the early part of this stay. His 58-year-old wife and 26-year-old daughter were openly anxious and would seek out the nurse on every shift to ask about his condition. The nurses' explanation to the family varied widely as the patient's condition changed. The differences were heightened for the family because there was little communication between the nurses as to what had been said on the previous day or previous shift. The patient's wife and daughter became increasingly anxious and sought out the nursing staff even more frequently. The head nurse became aware of the situation, met with the family, and discovered the problem of varying and conflicting information. A decision was made to assign a nurse on each shift to care for the patient for the rest of his stay instead of assigning a new nurse each day, and to have the nurse coming on duty at shift change be briefed by the off-going nurses as to what the family had been told. As soon as the nurses were consistent about information shared with the family, there was a prompt and marked decrease in anxiety in both wife and daughter. The agitated, frantic collaring of random nurses in the hallway stopped and the family became more supportive of the patient.

Negative Attitudes of Nurses to Families

Sometimes nurses can form attitudes about family members that can be a source of difficulty. These attitudes can grow from a feeling of which the nurses may only partially be conscious, or sometimes not conscious at all. The family members' age, sex, dress, demeanor, or appearance may trigger feelings in the nurse that can run the gamut from suspiciousness, dislike, antagonism, and fear to strong, positive feelings such as affection and admiration. Occasionally these feelings may develop before the nurse has gathered adequate data on the family member's interaction with the patient.

A 68-year-old male was transferred to the MICU from acute medicine after developing ECG changes. His diagnosis was to Rule Out MI. His wife was 66 years old and had chronic leukemia. Before the nursing staff had a chance to meet the patient's wife, the patient's 33-year-old son poured out a story of concern about his mother's "bad effect" on his father. As he described his mother as hyperactive, constantly talking, questioning, and moving aimlessly about, she was heard shouting loudly, demanding to see the patient. The nurses' initial contact with the patient's wife was colored by the information given by the patient's son. The nurse spent most of this initial meeting explaining why the patient could not be visited at the moment. The nurse formed her primary alliance with the son and together they decided on limiting the patient's wife's visiting to the "regular" visiting times, while the son had access to the patient at any time he came to the hospital, ostensibly because of his working hours. The nurse-son alliance kept the nursing staff at a considerable distance from the wife, who viewed the nurses with understandable open hostility. The patient did not appear to react unfavorably to his wife's visits, even though she did behave in the ways described by her son. For the remainder of the patient's stay on the MICU, there was friction and unpleasantness in interactions between the wife and the nursing staff. After the patient was transferred off the MICU, his wife returned to angrily accuse the staff of not sending all the patient's clothes with him to his new room.

APPROACHES TO DEALING WITH FAMILIES

It is in the clinical areas where the problems involving family members surface so forcefully that the nurse becomes aware—often painfully, angrily, and defensively—of the importance of the family member in the total treatment situation. There are a number of approaches that can be utilized to maximize the beneficial potentials in the patient/family/nurse interaction. These approaches are as follows:

1. Architectural
2. Administrative
3. Individual approaches to nurse/patient/family relationships
4. Group approaches to family members of ICU patients

Architectural

Architectural approaches to optimizing family member participation during a patient's ICU stay involve developing a physical environment on the ICU that allows for frequent family visiting, with reasonable privacy and, at the same time, the necessary nursing surveillance of the patient. The second part of the architectural approach is the development of ICU waiting rooms that are comfortable and as attractive as possible. Couches large enough to allow an adult to stretch out are especially important because family members often spend the night in the waiting room. An area where the nurse and physician can talk with families in privacy is needed.

Administrative

Administrative approaches to maximizing family participation deal primarily with regulating access to the patient; e.g., visiting hours. ICUs, early in their history, had very restrictive visiting policies. Visits of five to ten minutes every hour, or fifteen minutes every three hours, were not uncommon. In most ICUs where patients are in single rooms, there is very little reason for not having visiting hours on the ICU that are similar to those of the rest of the hospital's general nursing divisions. On a well-designed ICU, it should be possible for family members to spend reasonable amounts of time with the patient. At the same time, it is clear that the nursing personnel need to develop good channels of communication with the family members about visiting so that they can have the family members stay out of the room in order to: (1) carry out nursing procedures; (2) give patients necessary rest; and (3) interrupt potentially harmful patient/family interactions. This approach to visiting policy clearly places more responsibility with the nurse in regulating family access to the patient. Nurses respond to such arrangements with ambivalent feelings. Nurses with this responsibility go through shifts in attitudes from times when they are extremely liberal about allowing family access to the patient to periods when they make very restrictive interpretations of visiting regulations. Often, the shift in a nurse's attitude grows out of some unpleasant interaction with the family member about visiting (perhaps the family member was uncooperative when the nurse asked the family member to leave), or the nurse might be caught up in the middle of a hostile interaction involving patient, family member, and nurse.

Recognizing that there are times of increased stress on the nurses on units with more liberal interpretations of visiting, it is also clear that a flexible system offers much, both to patient and family. When visiting times are longer, often the family member is more willing to leave the hospital and go home for reasonable periods of time rather than spend long hours in the waiting room or pacing the halls between brief visiting periods.

Individual Nurse Contacts with Family Members

In the long run the most effective involvement with family members will grow out of the rapport developed between the individual nurse and the family. This is especially true, and also more easily attained, when the patients stay on the ICU longer than the usual four or five days. While some nurses have therapeutic personalities that permit them to quickly develop rapport with families, even naturally talented nurses often need help in working out a specific problem with a family. Almost all nurses benefit from in-service training programs that teach them techniques to: (1) better understand their relationship with families; and (2) cope with situations that evolve with family members.

Group Approaches to Families

A program of regular group meetings for family members in the ICU waiting room is particularly useful at the beginning of the ICU experience, when the crisis is often most intense for the family and when there is much information about the ICU that needs to be shared with the family. The group setting offers the opportunity to: (1) introduce the family members to key nursing and social work personnel in the hospital; (2) quickly familiarize and orient the family to ICU rules; (3) describe ICU functions and operation; (4) provide a channel of communication between family members and ICU nursing staff; and (5) utilize group dynamics for support for the family members during the time their relative is in the ICU.

STARTING A WAITING GROUP FOR FAMILIES

Description of the MICU

The MICU in the Jewish Hospital of St. Louis is a fifteen-bed unit. All beds have the capability of cardiac arrythmia monitoring. Patients are admitted to the MICU for a variety of reasons, but chest pain, myocardial infarction, respiratory distress, cardiac arrest, and respiratory arrest account for most of the admissions. All nursing personnel are registered nurses. All the nurses working on the unit have completed a three-week critical care course. The course is an intensive and thorough review of cardiac and pulmonary physiology and anatomy, blood chemistries, interpretation of cardiac arrythmias, and the use of specialized equipment such as ventilators and Swan-Ganz catheters. There is also a section of the course devoted to teaching patients and families about heart attack or chronic obstructive pulmonary disease and another section devoted to psychological factors involved in ICU nursing. The majority of the nurses work ten hours a day, four days a week. The head nurse works eight hours a day, for five days a week, in order to increase availability and communication. During the day shift, there are usually eight to nine nurses, one secretary, and one equipment orderly. One of the nurses is assigned to the monitors for the entire day and another nurse serves as charge nurse. Evening and night staffing consist of seven nurses and one unit secretary. An intern is always present on the MICU and a resident is either present or close by at all times. In addition, regular rounds are made by the cardiology and pulmonary departments together with the house staff and nursing staff, and rounds with other departments are made as necessary. There is a weekly meeting with a psychiatrist so that the nurses on the ICU can discuss psychological problems that occur in their work on the unit. In addition, regular staff meetings are held by the head nurse.

The Development of Meetings with Family Members and Friends of ICU Patients

Interactions of nurse/patient/family member had been a frequent focus of discussion in the regular consultation conference with the psychiatrist on this unit over a period of four years. After a number of weekly meetings in which the focus had been problems growing out of relationships with family members, the consultant psychiatrist suggested that regular meetings be established in the waiting room with family members in an effort to begin early, maximally beneficial, therapeutic contact with family members. The idea was quickly acted on by the head nurse of the unit, who had become aware of the problems growing out of family relationships. There were initial discussions between the head nurse and the psychiatrist about the form and content of group meetings for family members, and the psychiatrist agreed to act as supervisor of the meetings in the initial stages. A mutual decision was reached to involve a member of the social service department in the meetings. Two social workers were designated to participate in the project, one of whom was a student completing field work at the hospital and the other a full-time graduate social worker.

Initially it was decided to hold the meetings weekly at 1:30 p.m., a half hour before regular visiting hours on the MICU.

The meeting place was the waiting room. It was chosen for the convenience of the family and also for the largest possible attendance. A sign was placed in the waiting room announcing the time and date of the meeting. In order to facilitate continuity of the meetings, an assistant head nurse was also enlisted in the project to act as a co-leader of the group when the head nurse was not available.

The Format of the Meeting

The head nurse and the social worker begin the meeting by introducing themselves to the family members and friends in the waiting room. The head nurse then explains that the purpose of the meeting is to help relatives and friends cope with the difficult situation growing out of the illness of their family member who has been hospitalized on the MICU. The nurse goes on to explain the physical layout of the MICU. She describes the number of beds, the types of patients admitted, and what the monitors do. She also describes the physician staffing of the unit. She explains that the nurses on the unit have been specially trained to work with very sick patients. She discusses visiting hours and the position that the unit adopts to exceptions to visiting hours. She explains that more visiting time is possible if it is felt to be needed, but that visitors may be asked to leave at any time, even during regular visiting hours and for reasons other than the condition of their patient-family member.

The social worker also makes an introductory statement. This statement again emphasizes that the staff of the hospital recognizes the crisis for both patient and family growing out of admission to the ICU. The social worker discusses a number of common concerns that are frequently experienced by relatives and friends in the waiting room. There is a recognition that people in the waiting room often talk about their mutual problems. The group is told that the Social Service Department is available without charge to all family members and friends of the patient on an individual basis to discuss any aspect of either the acute illness or the recovery phase. Both co-leaders invite questions and comments. The meeting usually lasts 20 to 30 minutes.

Description of the Meetings

Attendance at the meetings depends, to a great extent, on the number of patients on the ICU on a given day. It is usual for there to be a group of eight to twelve people in the waiting room at the time of the meetings. There have been as many as twenty and, on a few occasions, there have been no people present when the meetings were scheduled. Because the average stay on the unit is short (about five days), most family members and friends participate in only one session of the ICU waiting room group. It is typical for the group to be rather quiet and subdued, although, at times, there have been one or two outspoken and angry people in the group. There is a high level of anxiety and depression that is quite palpable. Generally, there is some reticence in asking questions or presenting problems to the leaders of the group. Initially, one or two relatives tended to dominate the sessions by asking questions while the rest of the group would sit quietly, listening intently. The quiet "observers" often had high levels of anxiety that became apparent during the interchanges that developed during the course of the meeting. After the initial meetings, when it became clear that this was a typical pattern, the group leaders embarked on a course of action that was designed to involve everyone in the group, at least in some minimal way. This has been accomplished by having one of the leaders (the MICU head nurse) address each person in the room individually and ask which ICU patient they were visiting and how they were related to the patient. This method was especially useful to the head nurse because she was then able to rather quickly identify the patient, the patient's illness, length of stay, and any special problems the patient had presented.

The first meeting turned out to be rather typical for the waiting room group. After the initial introductions by head nurse and social worker, a 40-year-old black man began to express concern about finding babysitters for his young children. The man was the husband of a 40-year-old woman who had suffered severe brain damage following surgery and was terminally ill. The couple had nine children, some quite young. The social worker responded to the questions by being supportive about his concerns for the children and by talking with him about a referral to a community resource where home helper service could be obtained. The social worker also saw the husband after the meeting and worked out a short-term plan with him for having family members help in the crisis until more definite arrangements for the children would be worked out.

At the first meeting, several other questions were asked that turned out to be recurrent ones, asked in nearly every subsequent meeting. The first of these involved concern about what would happen to the patient after discharge from the ICU. Family members asking this kind of question were frequently able to express their anxiety about what they saw as the precarious state of the patient and the tension they felt because of the tubes, wires, and other mechanical support systems which, to them, emphasized the patient's helplessness and the threat of the illness to the patient's life. The question about the transfer from the ICU most often carried with it the concern that the patient would not receive as good care on the regular nursing division and sometimes expressed the ambivalence of the family about the good care received by their patient on the ICU and the anxiety aroused by the treatment "hardware."

The second question that became a regular feature of the meetings concerned cardiac catheterization. The ICU head nurse responded to this by providing detailed and specific information about the procedure and by allowing the family members to ventilate their anxiety—usually in the form of additional questions.

The third issue that frequently surfaced in the meeting was concern about caring for the patient at home. This often grew out of the question mentioned above about transfer off the ICU to a regular nursing division. It reflected many of the same anxieties and ambivalences that family members felt about their sick relative. These questions often became quite specific and touched on diet, exercise, medication, home nursing service, etc. The frequency of this question underlined its usefulness as a coping mechanism and as a vehicle for expressing anxiety. At times it was asked by a family member very early in a patient's stay when the medical situation was still a crisis or the immediate outcome unclear. Those questioners were using the question to deflect their attention from the still unresolved medical crisis and to reassure themselves that "their" patient would indeed be coming home.

At other times this question came from a family member whose ill relative was out of danger. The questioners in this situation were more often preoccupied with the increase in responsibilities. They were anticipating and expressing anxiety about these, and either overtly or covertly requesting help and support. Efforts would be made in the group to identify this as a common concern of family members, to focus on the individual nature of all of the rehabilitation programs, and to emphasize that the hospital had specific teaching and rehabilitation programs for heart attack and chronic pulmonary disease patients, which included family members and which began as soon as the patient was able to cooperate in the program (most often on the ICU and frequently completed on the regular nursing division to which the patient would be transferred from the ICU).

Guilt feelings would regularly surface in the meetings. These would usually take the form of questions about what "caused" heart attacks. Oftentimes the family member presenting this question would append to it some comment that indicated they were concerned that they may have done something that was responsible for the heart attack. These questions would sometimes reflect an undercurrent of anger that the family felt toward the patient. This was especially so when the questioners would emphasize the patient's behavior in ignoring risks, in not following the physician's advice or the family advice, eating or exercising imprudently, smoking too much, failing to relax or to take vacations, etc.

The leaders expressed interest in questions of this type, but avoided making any comments that would increase the guilt or blame for either the patient or the family member. Sometimes they indicated that they would try to get more information about specific aspects of questions like these and discuss them with the family member.

Over and over again, it became apparent that the relatives and friends present were using specific questions to both express and cope with the anxiety they were experiencing. It was unusual for relatives to talk openly and directly about issues such as whether the patient would live or die or about their feelings if the patient's condition became hopeless. Clearly, it was easier for them to ask what bubbles meant in the IV bottle, what normal ECG patterns were like, and under what circumstances cardiologists were called for consultation. The effort of the group leaders to involve the quiet members in the group was an important turning point in their ability to make the meetings more helpful. It often served to increase rapport with the family and make a better relationship between the family and those nurses providing care for the patient. In addition, this more active role provided direct help to some families. For example, the questioning of a relative in the waiting room, who had not asked any questions during the meeting, revealed that this relative had been sleeping in the waiting room for several nights. She had come from a small town some distance from the hospital and was not familiar with the city. The social worker was able to help find a hotel close to the hospital that had special rates for family members of patients.

Another quiet relative was the husband of a woman who had returned to the ICU for the third time in less than a year, with severe, multiple cardiac and respiratory problems. The head nurse recognized that the man looked familiar and said so. He then began to talk, not only about his wife's illness, which had been a very lengthy one, but the fact that he, too, was ill with hypertension. He revealed that he was on medicine but had not been taking his medicine regularly. The head nurse was supportive of him but also gave him some simple instructions about the importance of regularly taking antihypertension medication. However, the most critical part of this interchange was that the nurse recognized that the man was reaching out for help for himself—that he was under considerable strain because of his wife's lengthy hospitalization and because of his growing awareness that this hospitalization would end with his wife's death.

The recognition of his anxiety and the offer of support turned out to have an immediate short-term benefit. A few days after the meeting, the man's wife had a respiratory arrest and her condition became critical. The head nurse talked with the husband about the deterioration in his wife's condition and the contact established earlier made her communication with him more effective.

On a couple of occasions, people have been repeat members of the group. In each of these instances, the initial contact in the group has proved to be helpful in quickly establishing rapport.

It was characteristic of the meetings for at least one member of the group to voice support and confidence in the nurses and to praise the help the unit nurses were giving the patients and the families. On rare occasions, a member of the group openly voiced hostility. The first time this occurred was soon after the start of the meetings, when the wife of a patient denounced the social service department for failing to provide financial assistance. The woman's anger grew out of feeling trapped by her husband's illness and without any support. Her verbalized complaints were that, while some people seemed to offer help, help was not forthcoming. In contact prior to the meeting, the woman had been referred to a community resource to help her deal with a financial problem. She had rejected the referral angrily and was using anger in the meeting to help ward off some of her feelings of helplessness. This interaction, which occurred early in the meetings, was dealt with defensively by the co-leaders, who pointed out times when the social service department had been helpful to people who had been members of the ICU waiting room group. This response represented an expression of leader anxiety and a need for the co-leaders to protect one another when negative or critical feelings were expressed. Since that time, the leaders have been more able to tolerate expressions of hostility and criticism, when they are voiced, without being defensive and have tried to view these interactions as a special kind of coping mechanism that family members may exhibit when under great stress.

It was mentioned earlier that there were one or two meetings at which no family members were present. They both occurred in the second month of the waiting room group meetings. The meeting time was moved to 1:40 p.m., which was 10 minutes closer to the 2:00 p.m. start of visiting hours. This change in time has resulted in generally better attendance.

The meetings appear to be useful, although the usefulness is difficult to measure quantitatively. The ICU waiting room meeting has opened a communication channel between the family and key people on the hospital team. Frequently, after the meeting, families express gratitude that the "hospital cares about us." The meeting often provides useful information for the head nurse, which helps the nursing staff understand the family's position in relation to the sick family member. In one group, a family expressed concern about their 90-year-old mother, who had specifically told them prior to her illness that she wanted no resuscitation or mechanical devices to sustain her life if she ever became seriously ill. At that point, their mother was on a ventilator and was also being treated very vigorously by the medical team. The family felt guilty and anxious because they had not been able to tell the physicians about their mother's request and had not been able to make clear what their wishes were about their mother's treatment. In the meeting, they asked the head nurse for help with this. They voiced their guilt about having let their mother down. They talked about how their mother, who was at that time still aware of what was going on around her, would grimace and turn away from them when they came to visit her. The head nurse empathized with the difficult situation and encouraged them to talk more to her. After they had shared more of their feelings about it, the nurse arranged for them to talk with the physician responsible for their mother's care. The physician, armed with the information from the head nurse, was able to outline more clearly the options and consequences of the options to the family.

The ICU waiting room group, at this point, appears to be a viable, useful way of providing help to family members during a crisis. It is an opportunity to provide an important element and support system for the families' critical time and it offers the opportunity to enhance the rapport of the family with the nursing staff in ways that ultimately benefit patient care.

GUIDELINES FOR STARTING AN ICU WAITING ROOM GROUP

The Setting, Form, and Structure

FREQUENCY

A group that meets two or three times a week offers maximal support to the waiting room community, allows two or three contacts with relatives and visitors, provides an opportunity for greater expression of concerns, and gives the natural phenomenon of group support a chance to begin to function. If meetings at this frequency are not possible, a once-a-week format is workable, though not ideal.

TIME

Set the meeting time to begin 15 to 20 minutes before a regular visiting period on the ICU. A visiting period in the middle of the day is usually the one with the largest number of visitors and largest attendance. Set a definite time to end the meeting and stick to that time. In order to avoid resentment or anger on the part of the visitors, the time of the meeting should not intrude on visiting hours.

The leaders of the group should arrive at the meeting place about five minutes before the group. In addition, one of the group leaders should check in the patients' rooms to remind any relatives who are visiting that the meeting is to begin and to invite them to join.

PLACE

The meeting is best held in the waiting room itself, provided that there is room for the visitors to sit comfortably and that there is a reasonable absence of interruptions from traffic and the movement of people who have nothing to do with the meeting.

ANNOUNCING THE MEETING

Try to make all of the visiting family members aware of the meeting. A sign can be placed in the waiting room, which briefly identifies and describes the meeting and gives the time and place. In addition, a brief written description of the ICU waiting room group can be included in a brochure from the hospital and the ICU that is given to family members who visit. Finally, the nursing staff, in their individual contacts with the families, should make sure that family members know about the existence of the ICU waiting room group.

Staffing of the ICU Meeting

LEADER QUALIFICATIONS

Since the issues raised in the ICU waiting room tend to be rather wide-ranging, it is valuable to have co-leaders—a nurse and a social worker. The nurse should have specific knowledge of the patients on the unit and be thoroughly grounded in all the clinical and administrative matters related to the operation of the unit. Nurse specialists with advanced training in patient education and/or group dynamics are especially valuable as co-leaders of an ICU waiting room group. However, when nurses with this specialized background are not available, it is still possible to have an interested and knowledgeable nurse serve as a satisfactory leader provided she receives support from the other co-leaders and provided adequate consultation is available.

The other co-leader of the ICU waiting room group is one who ideally has knowledge and training in dealing with the social and psychological problems growing out of hospitalization for acute and chronic serious illness, who has a thorough and working knowledge of the hospital and community resources, and who has theoretical knowledge and practical experience in leading and working with groups.

SUPERVISION

It is useful to have a specialist in group dynamics meet regularly with the co-leaders of the group at intervals of two to three weeks (and even more frequently in the early phases of the group) to discuss the way the group is going, to help the co-leaders deal with problems they are facing in the group, to help with the training of the group leaders, and to act as a resource for these leaders.

Summaries should be made by the co-leaders after each meeting. It is often valuable for each co-leader to write his or her own summary of the meeting and later to pool these summaries as they discuss the meeting. Summaries of the meetings are also valuable when consultation is requested by the co-leaders. These summaries give the co-leaders a chance to compare the course of the meeting from session to session, to identify recurring themes, and to evaluate their own performances.

PLANNING AND COORDINATION

It is valuable in the early stages of the ICU group meetings for the co-leaders to meet briefly before the meeting. The purpose of this is to give the nurse, who usually has much more familiarity with current problems, a chance to alert the co-leader to any important matters that she thinks may possibly come up in the meeting. This briefing might involve a short description of the current patient population, a quick summary of any significant interactions among visitors, patients, and nursing staff on the unit, or any unusual events on the unit that may have had repercussions in the waiting room community, etc. It is also valuable for the co-leaders to meet immediately after the group to share their impressions of how the meeting went and to do a quick critique and evaluation.

Content and Process

OPENING STATEMENTS

Since the ICU waiting room turnover is so rapid, it is important that both leaders give a short and precise summary with specific information that describes: (a) the ICU; (b) the co-leader's areas of expertise; and (c) the kinds of help and information the co-leaders can provide. The co-leaders should be clear and specific and use non-technical language in their initial introduction. Both introductions should focus on the purpose of the group—which is to help, support, and inform family and friends who visit patients on the ICU.

ANSWERING QUESTIONS

Since the usual form of exchange in the waiting room group is question and answer, the leaders should try to provide specific and direct answers to questions where is is possible. However, the leaders should also be aware that the questions often are expressions of some underlying feeling state, and the questions may represent some type of coping effort by the questioner.

The co-leaders should be aware of the need most people in the group will have for some sort of support and comfort and should be prepared to give it. The giving of support, in this sense, includes providing specific information and identifying resources in the hospital or the community to help the patient and family with problems, and also includes the empathic identification of feeling states in the people in the group.

The co-leaders should recognize that there will be many questions that they cannot answer. It is important that the co-leaders establish a direct and honest relationship with the group. They should be able to be candid about questions they cannot answer. They should also make it clear that, where there is some question that they cannot answer, they will either try to find the answer or else direct the questioner to a resource where the answer can be obtained.

AWARENESS OF FEELINGS OF FAMILIES

Co-leaders should be aware of the high level of anxiety and depression that permeates the ICU waiting room. The leader should be aware that people will present common concerns that reflect their anxiety, tension, and depression in a number of ways, some of which may be indirect. It is important that the leaders treat all communicatons as important pieces of information and respond to them in that framework.

The co-leaders should be tolerant of expressions of feeling in the group. At times, there will be angry, complaining, or discouraged people in the ICU waiting room group. It is generally a better tactic to accept any angry statements or criticism without fighting back or feeling injured. Where explanations can be made in response to angry or critical remarks, they should be made in nondefensive ways—if possible, with the emphasis on clarification, information exchange, and acceptance of the feelings expressed.

DEVELOPING GROUP PROCESS

The co-leaders should allow a natural group process to develop in the group. The co-leaders should be aware that the group members, at times, will be able to support themselves, that sometimes other group members will have answers to questions, and that they will be able to provide the answers in ways that will often be very reassuring and helpful. The co-leaders should understand that they are not the only sources of information within the group and that the shared experience of other group members is an important element that needs to be exploited to make the group function optimally.

LEADER ACTIVITY

The group co-leaders should generally adopt an active role within the meeting. When the group is slow in starting or there appear to be no questions forthcoming, a useful way of breaking through initial resistance is for one of the leaders to "make the rounds" of the group by asking the people in the ICU group their names, whom they are visiting, how long their relative has been a patient, etc.

AWARENESS OF FEELINGS OF LEADERS

The co-leaders should be aware of their own sensitivity to the issues raised in the ICU waiting room group. It is important that the leaders try to identify their own areas of sensitivity and vulnerability. It is also important that the leaders should recognize that they need not automatically go to the defense of their co-leader if some anger or criticism is directed to the co-leader. Each leader should recognize her own autonomy and the sense of independence that she has as a leader and that her colleague, as co-leader, also has. Leaders should recognize that the ICU meeting may be only a beginning or jumping off point for work with an individual family and that, in many cases, some individualized contact with the family may be necessary outside the ICU meeting.

SHARING INFORMATION

The leaders should focus as much as possible on the opportunity to quickly and directly share information with the people in the group and to recognize that sharing of information and providing answers to questions often have a very quick anxiety-reducing effect. The group leaders willl become aware, through questioning, that there are many myths and misconceptions that grow up in and around the waiting room and that providing accurate information is one way of helping to deal with some of those myths and misconceptions.

CONTACT WITH PHYSICIANS

Keep the physicians who work on the unit aware of the ICU meetings. Make sure that the physicians know the kind of information that is given to the families at the meetings. Also try to share with the physicians relevant information that grows out of the ICU meetings.

CONTACT WITH NURSES

Make sure all the nurses in the ICU know about the meetings. It is valuable to share material from the meetings with nurses in nurses' report, so that they can make the best use of the information that comes from the meetings in their more individualized work with patients and family.

CLOSING AND FOLLOW-UP

The co-leaders should make sure that the relatives and visitors have specific instructions about how they can reach each of the co-leaders after the meetings for any additional questions, clarification, or information.

SUMMARY

Families can play critical roles in the course of the patient's illness by affecting the patient's emotional state or the state of the nurses who care for the patient. Families also have needs, as human beings experiencing great stress, that in part become the concern of the ICU nurses. Once the importance of the family role is recognized, steps can be taken to offer appropriate services. ICU waiting rooms need to be designed with the family of the ICU patient in mind. Both comfort and some degree of privacy are highly desirable. Flexible visiting hours are also most often useful and in the best interests of the patient, family, and nursing staff, even though there can be many special exceptions to this general rule. Families, nurses, and patients interact in a complex and wide variety of ways, and the ICU nurse must be ready to work to understand as thoroughly as possible how the family interaction is affecting the patient and her professional role with the patient.

Finally, the waiting room community itself, with proper leadership, can become a therapeutic instrumentality. Waiting room groups can be formed and led by nurses and other professionals with group leadership training. A waiting room group is described in detail and suggestions are made on how such groups can be formed.

REFERENCES

1. Michaels D: Too Much in Need of Support to Give Any. Am J Nurs 71: 1932–1935, 1971

2. West N: Stresses Associated with ICU's Affect Patient, Families, Staff. Hosp 49: 362–376, 1975

3. Ryan MA: Helping the Family Cope with a Cardiac Arrest, Nurs 74: 80–81, 1974

4. Cooper C: The Waiting Room. Am J Nurs 76: 273, 1976

5. Skelton M, Dominian J. Psychological Stress in Wives of Patients with Myocardial Infarction. Brit Med J 8: 101–103, 1973

CHAPTER 15

*Psychiatric Consultation with MICU Nurses: The Consultation Conference as a Working Group**

Nathan M. Simon and Suzanne Whiteley

The events described in this article took place in the course of a year in which a group of remarkable nurses on a Medical Intensive Care Unit (MICU) established a consultation conference with a psychoanalyst. The chapter will describe how it developed and changed. It is also an account of the discovery that the participants in the conference were "talking prose," that is, doing something rather elegant with little self-consciousness. It will also touch on some issues that are related to bringing a research focus into a consultation setting.

The authors' search of literature revealed ten papers that discussed the psychological aspects of the intensive-care unit (ICU) as they relate to the nursing staff.[1–10] These papers have several characteristics in common: (1) they mostly describe Surgical Intensive Care Units (SICU) or mixed units, not MICU; (2) all comment at length about the psychological problems and hazards of working on such units; (3) there is a similarity of views about the toll taken by these hazards; and (4) none describes any efforts to help the nurses deal with the psychological stresses of ICU work. A quote from Hay and Oken[8] gives the flavor of many of these papers. "A stranger on entering an ICU is at once bombarded with a massive array of sensory stimuli, some emotionally neutral but many highly charged. Initially the greatest impact comes from the intricate machinery with its flashing lights, buzzing and beeping

*Reproduced with permission from Heart & Lung 6: 497–504, 1977; copyrighted by The C. V. Mosby Company, St. Louis, Missouri, U.S.A.

monitors, gurgling suction pumps and whooshing respirators. Simultaneously one sees many people rushing around busily performing life-saving tasks. The atmosphere is not unlike that of a tension-charged strategic war bunker. One becomes aware of desperately ill, sick and injured human beings and they are hooked up to the machinery. And in addition to the mechanical stimuli, one can discern moaning, crying, screaming and the last gasps of life. Sights of blood, vomitus, excreta, exposed genitalia, multilated and wasted bodies, and unconscious and helpless people assault the sensibilities. Many are neither alive nor dead. Most have tubes in every orifice. Their sounds and action or inaction are almost inhuman."

THE SETTING

The conference grew out of an invitation from the nurses to the senior author to participate with them in the conference. They were depressed about a series of events that had occurred in the MICU and were also concerned that they were becoming insensitive to the patients as people. A joint decision was reached to meet for one hour every two weeks and to center discussions around specific problems related to patients.

The Jewish Hospital MICU is a second-generation MICU and quite different from the one described above. It has 15 beds, each in private rooms arranged on a long hall. The rooms are well-insulated for noise. Each has a window that opens to the outside. The colors are subdued, neutral tones. It is a quiet place. People are visible around the unit, but only rarely look as if they are involved in any great crisis—even though crises occur constantly. There is a subdued, modulated, and well-controlled atmosphere about the place. Of the 15 beds, four are reserved for the pulmonary service. The bulk of the admissions to the Jewish Hospital MICU are patients with acute myocardial infarctions or those for whom myocardial infarctions are being ruled out. The average stay on the unit is a little over five days. The unit was staffed at that time with 30 nurses and eight monitor technicians. Most of the nurses are young women (there are two men), but six of the 24 on whom we have data are over 30 years of age. Fifteen of them have worked on the unit for over a year. Most of them are RNs with some training beyond the RN degree.

There are two interns and one resident assigned full-time and a large teaching staff with part-time assignments in the MICU. There are two full-time internists who divide clinical and administrative responsibilities. There is a good deal of tension over who actually has control over the patients. Much of that tension is submerged or ignored, but it erupts sporadically in the course of work. The private physicians feel that their patients are still "theirs," but they often complain about the limitations on who writes orders and what kinds of things are done. The interns, who write most of the orders, are often uncertain. Much buck-passing goes on about difficult decisions, with each level in the hierarchy (nurses, house staff, attending physicians) accusing the other of dodging the issues.

The nurses' working hours differ from the hours of those on the other nursing divisions, and this adds to the impression that the MICU is a "special" place. They work 10 hours a day, four days a week. The head nurse, who is administratively in charge of nursing staff, spends much of her time in patient care. The position of charge nurse is changed daily, and this job is assigned to all members of the nursing staff, including LPNs. A nurse on the unit will be assigned one very ill patient or two or three not-so-ill patients. During the day and evening shifts, there are about eight nurses and two monitor technicians on duty. The night shift has five RNs and two monitor technicians. In the months immediately preceding the conference, the unit was understaffed and there were many administrative problems. Tension was high and morale was quite low among the nurses.

Clinical problems complicated and contributed to the low morale. There were three people with chronic obstructive pulmonary diseases (COPD) on the unit for a very long time (two to three months). They all died. They were all machine-maintained for long periods of time. The issues of how much longer they were to be supported, why they were staying in the MICU, who was keeping them alive, and what the outcome would be were constantly in the air. It took a considerable toll of the nurses. The situation was complicated because, at that time, the nurses had little experience with the respiratory patients.

The nurses were frustrated, depressed, and angry. They had complained openly and bitterly about the work overload, the lack of adequate numbers of people to do the work, and the schedules. They felt their complaints were not listened to seriously.

THE INITIAL PHASE

The conference was scheduled every two weeks for an hour, but always ran longer. It was scheduled to take advantage of the overlap of personnel that occurred in midafternoon when both day and evening shifts were on the unit. On occasions, some people would come to the hospital on their days off to be part of the conference. Only two meetings were cancelled. There were from four to eight nurses present at the meetings.

At our first meeting, the nurses chose as the patient for discussion a young woman, 25 years old, who was a nurse and who had worked on a neurosurgical intensive-care unit. She had a spinal cord transection at the T-5 level. She was in the MICU because she had developed renal shutdown. She had been three months pregnant at the time of her injury while riding as a passenger with her husband on a motorcycle. This patient presented a host of complex emotional issues to nursing staff members who were virtually her twin sisters. They shared the same work, they were the same age, some of them were married about the same length of time, and one was pregnant. The nursing problem that was presented to the consultant very briefly was that she had been sleeping very poorly, crying out, and having nightmares. The consultant talked to the patient just prior to the conference. She spontaneously reported a recurrent dream. She was sitting on her husband's lap, she was well, they were being very affectionate with one another, and they were in the living room of their house. The visit lasted for about 20 minutes. We talked a little about the dream and about her injury. The nightmares stopped, and her sleep problems improved considerably. The dynamics of the patient are not the central issue here except to indicate the way the conference began.

There was a very active discussion at the first meeting. The first thing the consultant discovered was his naivete. The consultant had thought that much time would be spent in the beginning going over the "A-B-Cs" of observation and data collection. He learned immediately that his colleagues in the conference were a bright, sophisticated group of people who knew a great deal about how people felt. They were able to describe feelings and behavior in clear, understandable ways and showed a great skill in maintaining contact with people who were under great stress in very bad situations. They made very important observations and contributions to the conference from the beginning.

In the initial conferences, the consultant tried to get the nurses to talk about what they actually do and to say what they try to do. Effort was focused on having the nursing staff verbalize as much as they could and identify their feelings. The consultant wanted to reinforce the obvious interest that the nurses already had in observation and understanding and make sure that they could put this to use. The consultant used modified role playing that was as close to the reality of the situation as possible. Because the patients are cared for by many nurses, there was a wealth of complementary data.

The early meetings tended to be more structured by conscious choice on the part of the consultant. Such topics as the depressed patient who is demanding; or the patient who has given up; or the patient who is dying and clearly beyond help and often on a ventilator, were dealt with. Occasionally, in those early meetings, the consultant would give short lectures on personality dynamics, the coronary-prone personality, and depression and loss.

However, in each of the early meetings, the low morale of the staff and the current intrastaff problems and intraunit problems would surface. There were many complaints, both overt and subtle, about the hospital and nursing administration, the private doctors, the house staff, especially the interns, and the "bad" things that would happen when patients were sent to the regular medical and surgical nursing divisions. The elitism characteristic of specially trained, highly skilled, and somewhat physically isolated personnel who perform very dangerous tasks began to appear. The consultant indicated interest in hearing about these things, even though they would appear in flashes. Sometimes, in the longer discussions, people made efforts to modulate the critical or unpleasant things that were being said.

The meetings varied greatly in quality. Sometimes there was little interest, and energy and effort were required to find something to talk about. Others were vibrant, intense, and moving. The most moving parts of the meetings for the consultant were the ways the nurses were handling the situations they were describing and what they were able to do with their feelings. The consultant frequently took a very active role by clarifying issues, delineating preconscious content, and focusing on identifications, transference-like reactions, guilt, anger, and other feelings.

In the early meetings, we often talked about people with advanced COPD who were being maintained on a ventilator. Who was going to pull the plug? What was the sense of the patient's continuing to live, supported constantly by the ventilator? The nursing staff was angry with the interns, the private physicians, the full-time staff, the patients, and, of course, themselves. These meetings were often very intense. Ambivalent feelings about old people began to surface, along with concerns about death and dying.

In one meeting, a nurse became aware of a host of intense feelings that were aroused as she cared for a middle-aged man hospitalized for myocardial infarction. She found herself anxious, angry, and many times reluctant to go into the room to be with the patient. All of this was quite unusual for this young woman, who was one of the outstanding nurses on the unit. She presented the situation at a conference and openly voiced her difficulties in caring for the patient. The other nurses were quite surprised. All of them saw him as a rather routine patient who had not presented them with any particular problem. As she went on to talk, she became aware that the patient resembled her own father in many ways. He was the same age, looked somewhat like him, and had a family of young children very much like the nurse's own family. She was somewhat uncomfortable as she continued to talk and express these feelings and thoughts, but there was a good deal of support from the other nurses in the meeting and, by the end of the meeting, other nurses were talking of similar situations in which they had identified patients with important people in their lives and of the feelings that were aroused.

THE MIDPHASE

After about three months of regular meetings, the conferences began to change. Nurses were no longer choosing in advance specific patients for discussion. They were more comfortable and willing to see what would develop spontaneously. The consultant encouraged this by indicating a willingness to explore the concerns of the moment. The nurses would sometimes complain about the lack of structure and invite the consultant to return to the old format. At times, this appeared to the consultant (and was later confirmed by information from the nurses) to be an expression of resistance to the awareness of the complexity of feelings aroused spontaneously in earlier meetings. On other occasions, this represented: (1) a legitimate request for more organized presentation of material (especially when the preceding meeting was unsuccessful); (2) an expression of unavailability of energy after a tense and exhausting work shift; and (3) a vote of disagreement with some of the consultant's ideas.

While this fluctuating situation was going on in the meetings, the acceptance of the consultant as a competent professional was growing, as evidenced by the number of times nurses sought him out to talk about personal problems.

Another feature of this stage was a decision to allow the monitor technicians to attend the conferences. Two things accounted for this: (1) requests by a few technicians, who were genuinely interested, and by a few who saw their earlier exclusions as more evidence of their "second-class citizenship" in the hierarchy; and (2) nurses, who did not wish to attend, and who saw this as a way of sending a substitute.

The meetings during this period alternated between being resistant and intense. In some of the latter sessions, highly charged personal problems involving staff relationships surfaced. One of these sessions focused on sex. It began with a nurse asking about the sexual capacities of men who were quadraplegic. A quadraplegic man she was caring for often had erections while she was giving him his bed bath and often talked to her in very sexual terms. After the consultant had clarified the nurse's concern about being in a sexual situation, there was a very active discussion about the frequency with which sex came up in the care of their male patients. Their denial, uncertainty, embarrassment, anger, and surprise were discussed. The discussion moved then into the area of how patients were using open sexual behavior to help them deal with their illness and also to communicate with the nursing personnel. This issue was clarified fairly easily. The consultant then tried, without success, to move into the area of how the nurses themselves might be using their sexuality in interactions with the patients and staff. The nurses ignored the consultant's efforts to focus on this and continued to keep the discussion carefully within the bounds of what the patients were doing to the nurses. Most of the nurses felt that this was a highly successful session. The consultant in many ways agreed. However, it was clear that the efforts of the consultant to explore more anxiety-provoking areas and those areas considered to be more private by the nurses were resisted quite successfully.

There was another meeting about the same time that illustrated the same issue. This meeting began slowly with people having difficulty finding a topic they wished to discuss. After a few minutes of desultory talk, a nurse began talking in a seemingly casual way about cigarette smoking on the unit and the problems it created. When the subject was introduced, the focus was on the effect on the patients when staff members smoked on rounds. Later, it developed that many of the nurses were unhappy about their colleagues who smoked during nursing report time in a very small room used for that meeting.

As people began to talk more about this, two of the nursing staff, one man and one woman, ostentatiously lit cigarettes. The consultant made efforts to get the others to focus on the feelings that were being aroused as the discussion went on. However, there was a good deal of anger and much defensiveness on the part of almost everybody in the meeting and there was an inability to move into any area where the subject could be dealt with at a more adaptive level. One of the reasons this proved to be so difficult was that the smoking issue was being used as a vehicle to express feelings about several rather deep-seated splits among the nursing staff members on the unit that were seen as not openly discussable. This meeting was one which both the nursing staff and the consultant felt had been unsuccessful. Rather than reduce tensions, it served only to make things more tense.

Another meeting toward the end of this midphase of the consultation conference occurred on the last day that the head nurse worked on the unit. At that meeting, the resigning head nurse and two or three nurses who had been her severest critics were present. During the meeting, the consultant recognized that this was the head nurse's last day and invited her to talk about the situation and invited the others, too, to talk about the process of leaving and change. The resigning head nurse made a brave effort to talk about the problems of the past months. She used a good deal of denial and projection, but was trying to leave with some pride and without feeling a complete sense of defeat. The other nurses were uncomfortable, did not challenge her openly, and generally tended to leave her defenses alone.

The three meetings described above illustrate aspects of resistance that appeared during the midphase. Each served a variety of adaptive purposes for the group, and each indicated issues and feelings that could not be confronted directly.

The nursing staff welcomed the appointment of the new head nurse enthusiastically. She was an excellent nurse and was well liked by her colleagues. When she assumed her responsibilities, there was general improvement in morale on the unit. With this improvement, there was some shift in the subject matter at the consultation conferences, with the group again talking about individual cases and with fewer references to staff conflict.

THE LATE PHASE

The third phase in the evolution of the conference was characterized by informality, spontaneity, openness, and a high level of participation by the nursing staff. In one of these late-phase meetings, a nurse who had worked on a unit for a few months was discussing her response to an elderly woman patient, who had commented to her that the nurse would be alive the next day while she, the patient, would probably be dead. The patient died within a few days. The nurse was at first puzzled by the rather strange feelings she had about the woman's death, but, quite on her own and in a remarkable display of a psychological introspection, she was able to verbalize how angry she felt at the old woman who had tried to make her feel guilty during the last day or so in which the nurse had cared for her. She had been furious with the woman for her guilt-provoking efforts, had felt attacked by her, and then had felt guilty about her anger. This provided a springboard for a very active discussion about other guilt-provoking situations the nurses experienced with patients and also about the ambivalence and discomfort they felt when caught in situations where they were both angry and guilty about the anger.

Another session soon after this focused very painfully and poignantly on responses to helplessness. A 21-year-old man had been admitted to the unit with an illness that was characterized by a nectrotizing vasculitis. While he was in critical condition and bleeding profusely and while the medical staff was also quite clearly helpless to do anything about the rapid progression of his illness, the patient was conscious and terribly frightened about dying. He talked and cried and was terrorized by his illness. His father, who visited him during the few minutes allotted, talked to him about getting better and being brave. His wife, who was about the same age as the nurses, wept helplessly and had great difficulty being in the room with her husband. The nurses identified with the wife, were very angry with the father and with the doctors, and found that they themselves did not know how to respond to the patient when they had to care for him. The discussion focused on feelings of helplessness, the limits of what could be said, various ways in which support and comfort could be given nonverbally, and also the dangers of trying to reassure someone verbally when, indeed, neither the person trying to reassure nor the patient who is to be reassured can believe in what was being said. One of the nurses told how, after leaving work on the day she cared for this young man, she sat in her car and beat her hands against the dashboard until she felt some reduction of tension and anxiety. The discussion of this case took a couple of meetings, as some of the nurses who had not been present in the first session, but who had also cared for the patient, also felt a great need for some sort of opportunity to discuss their experiences in caring for him.

In the later sessions, the nurses began to shift to some of their own mistakes, while in earlier sessions, mistakes of private physicians, house staff, and administrators were favorite subjects. This was clearly an important turning point in the conference and indicated greater comfort on the part of the nurses in being able to be openly honest about issues where they might feel very vulnerable and subject to attack.

Another fruitful area of discussion that came up on a couple of occasions had to do with the nursing staff response to departures of other staff members. It occurred, for the first time, in a way that could be clearly identified when one of the nurses, who had worked on the unit five years, left to have a baby. She was a well-liked, extremely steady, hardworking, responsible nurse and had served as acting head nurse shortly before the conference was begun. Many people who knew her well felt her departure as a loss. There were depressed feelings that came up, at first seemingly unrelated to her departure, but the situation was quickly clarified. Several of the nurses were able to talk about their ambivalent feelings about their friend's departure.

The same situation occurred again when the "new" head nurse announced her resignation because her husband was moving to a new city. The subject matter was more easily identified by the nursing staff the second time because of the earlier experience. The session at which it first became an open issue was one in which a nurse began talking about what could be done to more easily integrate the new nursing staff into the working teams of the unit. However, because of the consultant's awareness of the head nurse's resignation, it was very easy to focus on concerns about changes on the unit, specifically about the head nurse's departure. Again, two or three very highly-charged and affect-laden meetings occurred, as the nursing staff made some effort to come to grips with a whole host of feelings occasioned by the coming departure of the head nurse.

There was one other major shift in the quality and character of the consultation conferences. After meeting for a year, the consultant suggested it would be valuable to write an article about the experience. The consultant had not thought about this when the conference began, but it was something that had been growing in his mind over the months as he met with the group. The consultant invited them to be part of the writing effort, asked for volunteers to help, and also asked the nurses to contribute ideas about what could go into the article itself. He invited the nurses to describe their participation, what they felt was important, and the way the conference affected the MICU. There was much enthusiasm initially about writing an article. However, these halcyon days soon ended.

In the meetings that followed, suspicious feelings were verbalized by many members of the nursing staff. They wondered whether the consultant had, in some ways, been "experimenting on them from the beginning." They wondered whether the consultant had been making notes about the meetings (which, to his regret, he had not been) and whether the idea for a "research project" had been important from the beginning in his interest in participating in the conference. In the sessions that followed, there was also a good deal of resentment and anger. The meetings were late in starting, attendance dropped precipitously, and cancellation of two meetings occurred during this time.

The nurses did draw up and distribute a six-page, 22-item questionnaire. Twenty-three of them—all of whom had attended at least one conference—completed the questionnaire. One of the nurses worked with the consultant in reviewing the responses and preparing and coauthoring the chapter.

The paper was read to and discussed by a group of 10 nurses prior to submission for publication. The suspiciousness about the consultant and also the feelings that were aroused by being "subjects" of a "research project" began to subside. Attendance picked up, and recent meetings have been characterized by a high level of functioning, with restoration of trust in the consultant. In addition, the nursing staff requested that the consultant meet with them more frequently and the meetings were increased to once a week. The research theme clearly became the vehicle that permitted open expression of negative and hostile transference feelings to the consultant, which had appeared previously only indirectly.

DISCUSSION

The authors' survey of the literature revealed a number of papers that acknowledged the rather special stresses to which nurses on ICU are subjected. None has reported a regular meeting like the one described in this paper. Almost all of the papers make suggestions about helping the nurses to cope with these stresses. Hay and Oken,[8] in their fine paper, suggested group meetings which would: (1) allow the nurses to express their hostility and gripes; (2) recognize the guilt, shame, anger, fear, and uncertainty that are accepted in shared experience; (3) provide an opportunity for abreacting; (4) allow for the sharing of innovative techniques in dealing with problems; (5) allow for recognition and acknowledgment of problems growing out of omnipotent fantasies; (6) recognize that mistakes are ubiquitous; and (7) provide a forum for constructing channels to enhance communication among the staff members.

Those of us who participated in this conference discovered that we were "talking prose." That is, without awareness of the suggestions made in the literature in which new options are to be given to the staff in helping them deal with a very difficult work situation, we quite innocently constructed a group meeting in which the things that were suggested by Hay and Oken[8] actually did transpire and were valuable. The conferences, as far as we can evaluate now, accomplished the things that were thought would accrue from the establishment of such group meetings.

The development of the meetings themselves was unremarkable as far as group process was concerned. There were clearly: (1) stages of initial, somewhat formal, and compliant acceptance of the meetings; (2) a period in which the meetings began to produce tensions and anxieties as feelings of the participants were stirred up; (3) a period of resistance and withdrawal as participants worked over issues such as the ability to trust the consultant and also trust their colleagues in the meetings; and finally (4) a stage of working through to a fairly high level of trust and confidence and a good deal of openness, freedom, and integrative participation in the meetings.

Meetings of this sort are representative of a group of phenomena obvious within both medicine and society as a whole. That is, there are some very simple and obvious things that can be done to help people deal with difficult situations. What is most surprising is how infrequently they are utilized. One of the remarkable things about this conference that quite clearly related to its successes was that the wish for the conference came from a small group of the nursing staff members. They provided a nucleus that made it possible to continue the conferences, they provided a positive feeling about the value of the conferences, and they allowed other nurses, who were less enthusiastic originally, to find out for themselves how it could be used. In addition, this consultation conference benefited from the consistent, steady support from the one full-time member of the Department of Medicine who was very enthusiastic about the conferences and initially encouraged the nurses. He was respected by all the nurses as a dedicated, highly competent physician who was committed to high-quality care for the patients and who was understanding and supportive of the nurses. While his support was low-key and subtle, it was clearly of great importance and helped counterbalance the highly ambivalent quality of the response of both the "first" head nurse and the nursing department of the hospital to the establishment of the conference. In retrospect, one wonders what would have happened to the conference had this quiet, but consistent, support not been available during the initial stages of the consultation conference.

Finally, this experience indicates the problems of introducing a research focus into what was originally not a research setting. Data collection, establishment of base lines, and identification of elements to be measured and changes that occurred are made extremely difficult when an attempt is made a year later to report on a complex process such as this conference. Notes after each meeting, regular evaluation of the nurses, and systematic analysis of the contents of the sessions related to the ward situation at the time would have been valuable. Offer and Sakhen[9] have demonstrated that it is possible to engage people in a research alliance, to keep them interested and involved over long periods of time, and to make the whole process of gathering data a consistent and systematic enterprise. The authors suggest to others who would embark upon such a conference that careful thought be given in advance to whether or not data from the conference are to be used for research. If such is an intention, the preparation for gathering data should be made prior to institution of the conference and the participants approached explicitly about the research focus.

It became clear from this experience that, when a research focus is introduced, the participants will have a very strong response to it. While initially there was high enthusiasm, this covered feelings that were quite different. The nurses were very disturbed by the rather sudden announcement that the consultant would consider their conference as a research activity. They became highly suspicious of the consultant's motives, and the conference developed a period of decompensation that lasted several weeks.

SUMMARY

A group of MICU nurses responded to a series of acute and chronic clinical and administrative stresses by establishing a consultation conference with a psychoanalyst. The evolution of the consultation conference into an ongoing working group is described. Its value as a modality to help deal with the special stresses of MICU nursing personnel is discussed. The problems of introducing a research focus into the conference were examined.

REFERENCES

1. Koumans AJR: Psychiatric Consultation in an Intensive Care Unit. JAMA 194: 633–637, 1965

2. Hammes HJ: Reflection on Intensive Care. Am J Nurs 68: 339–340, 1968

3. Kornfeld DS, Maxwell P, Momrow D: Psychological Hazards of Intensive Care Units—Nursing Care Aspects. Nurs Clin North Am 3: 41–45, 1968

4. Vreeland R, Ellis GL: Stresses on the Nurse in an Intensive Care Unit. JAMA 208: 332–334, 1969

5. Jones B: Inside the Coronary Care Unit. Am J Nurs 67: 2313–2320, 1967

6. Kornfeld DS: Psychiatric View of the Intensive Care Unit. Br J Med 115: 108–110, 1969

7. Gardam JED: Nursing Stresses in the Intensive Care Unit. JAMA 208: 2337–2338, 1969

8. Hay D, Oken D: The Psychological Stress of Intensive Care Unit Nursing. Psychos Med 34: 109–117, 1972

9. Cassem NH, Hackett TP: Sources of Tension for the CCU Nurse. Am J Nurs 72: 1426–1430, 1972

10. Gentry WD, Foster SB, Froehling S: Psychological Response to Situational Stress in Intensive and Nonintensive Nursing. Heart and Lung 1: 793–796, 1972

11. Offer D, Sakhen M: Research Alliance vs. Therapeutic Alliance: A Comparison. Am J Psych 123: 1519–1526, 1967

INDEX

D

E

F

G

H

I

J

L

M

N

O

P

Q

R

S

T

U

V

DATE DUE

GAYLORD			PRINTED IN U.S.A.